Nursing Knowledge Tree
An Initiative by CBS Nursing Division

Practical Record Book of

# Nursing Foundations

for BSc Nursing Students

*As per the Revised INC Syllabus (2021-22) for BSc Nursing*

**Second Edition**

**Amandeep Kaur**
*Associate Professor*
Institute of Nursing Education
Guru Teg Bahadur Sahib (C) Hospital
Ludhiana, Punjab

CBSPD
*Dedicated to Education*

**CBS Publishers & Distributors Pvt Ltd**

• New Delhi • Bengaluru • Chennai • Kochi • Kolkata • Lucknow • Mumbai
• Hyderabad • Jharkhand • Nagpur • Patna • Pune • Uttarakhand

Practical Record Book of
**Nursing Foundations**
for BSc Nursing Students

**ISBN: 978-93-90619-76-4**



**Reprint: 2025**

Second Edition: 2022

First Edition: 2019



Published by **Satish Kumar Jain** and produced by **Varun Jain** for

**CBS Publishers & Distributors Pvt Ltd**
4819/XI Prahlad Street, 24 Ansari Road, Daryaganj, New Delhi 110 002, India.
Ph: +91-11-23289259, 23266861, 23266867 Website: www.cbspd.com
Fax: 011-23243014
e-mail: delhi@cbspd.com; cbspubs@airtelmail.in.

***Corporate Office:*** 204 FIE, Industrial Area, Patparganj, Delhi 110 092
Ph: +91-11-4934 4934 Fax: 4934 4935
e-mail: feedback@cbspd.com; bhupesharora@cbspd.com

***Branches***

- **Bengaluru:** Seema House 2975, 17th Cross, K.R. Road, Banashankari 2nd Stage, Bengaluru 560 070, Karnataka
  Ph: +91-80-26771678/79 Fax: +91-80-26771680 e-mail: bangalore@cbspd.com
- **Chennai:** 7, Subbaraya Street, Shenoy Nagar, Chennai 600 030, Tamil Nadu
  Ph: +91-44-26680620, 26681266 Fax: +91-44-42032115 e-mail: chennai@cbspd.com
- **Kochi:** 68/1534, 35, 36-Power House Road, Opp. KSEB, Cochin-682018, Kochi, Kerala
  Ph: +91-484-4059061-65 Fax: +91-484-4059065 e-mail: kochi@cbspd.com
- **Kolkata:** Hind Ceramics Compound, 1st floor, 147, Nilganj Road, Belghoria, Kolkata-700056, West Bengal
  Ph: +033-2563-3055/56 e-mail: kolkata@cbspd.com
- **Lucknow:** Basement, Khushnuma Complex, 7-Meerabai Marg (Behind Jawahar Bhawan), Lucknow-226001, Uttar Pradesh
  Ph: +0522-4000032 e-mail: tiwari.lucknow@cbspd.com
- **Mumbai:** PWD Shed, Gala No. 25/26, Ramchandra Bhatt Marg, Next to J.J. Hospital Gate No. 2, Opp. Union Bank of India, Noor Baug, Mumbai-400009, Maharashtra
  Ph: +91-22-66661880/89 Fax: +91-22-24902342 e-mail: mumbai@cbspd.com

***Representatives***

- **Hyderabad** +91-9885175004
- **Nagpur** +91-9421945513
- **Pune** +91-9623451994
- **Jharkhand** +91-9811541605
- **Patna** +91-9334159340
- **Uttarakhand** +91-9716462459

***Printed at:*** *Rashtriya printers Delhi-110095*

## CBS Nursing Knowledge Tree

# Extends its Tribute to

# Florence Nightingale

*For glorifying the role of women as nurses,*
*For holding the title of "The Lady with the Lamp,"*
*For working tirelessly for humanity–*
*Florence Nightingale will always be*
*remembered for her*
*selfless and memorable services to the*
*human race.*

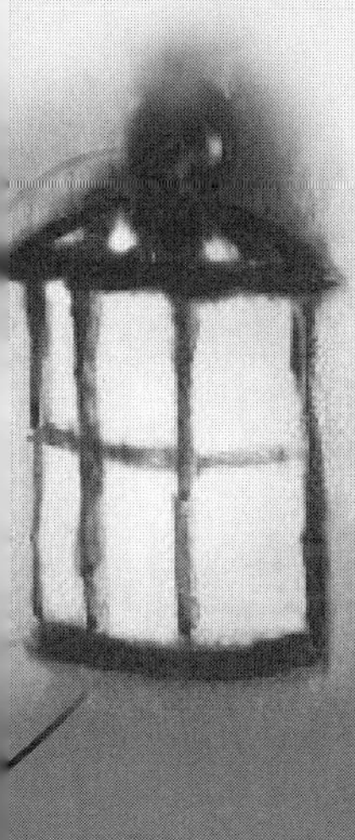

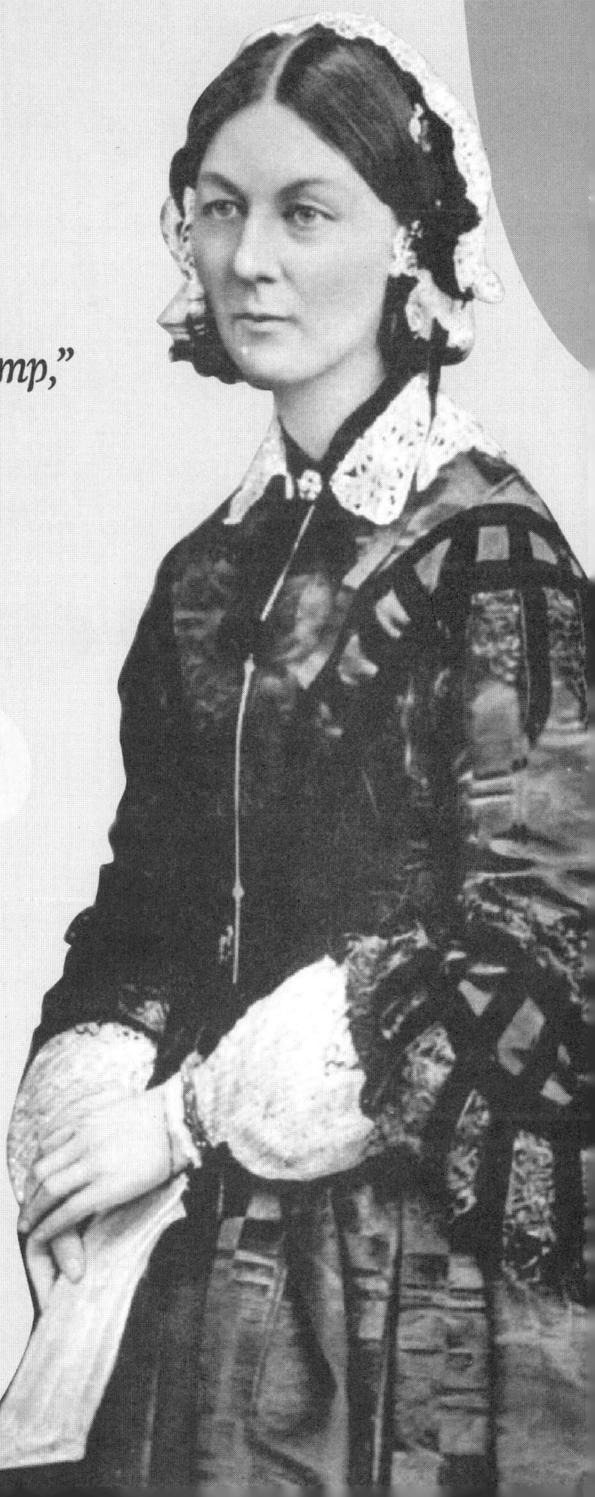

**Florence Nightingale**
**(May 1820 – August 1910)**

# Preface

Nursing assessment is the key component of nursing practice. It is a process of gathering information related to patient's physiological, psychological, sociological and spiritual status. The process is performed by a nurse. It is the first step in the nursing process which directs the rest of the process. It is a skill; the more you practice, the better you become.

This Practical Record Book of Nursing Foundations is intended to assist first-year Semester I & II BSc Nursing Students in their clinical requirements. The purpose of this record book is to improve the critical thinking and clinical skills of the budding student nurses.

This record book serves as a direction to nursing students to gather patient's health information, perform physical examination and provide comprehensive care to a patient. It clearly outlines the observations to be made by them. This book includes all the clinical criteria, i.e., history taking, general physical examination, nursing care plans, health talk and observation report, to be fulfilled during their first year of BSc Nursing course. Special attention has been given to provide a clear and concise presentation of content that can be easily understood by the students.

**Amandeep Kaur**

# Acknowledgments

*"He who has no faith in himself can never have faith in God."*

*—Guru Nanak Dev Ji*

I owe my sincere gratitude to the God for His unconditional grace and abundant blessings bestowed upon me throughout my life. I express my profound sense of gratitude and heartfelt thanks to all my teachers whom I see as a guiding force behind this work.

I extend my special thanks to **Mr Satish Kumar Jain** (Chairman) and **Mr Varun Jain** (Managing Director), M/s CBS Publishers and Distributors Pvt Ltd for their wholehearted support in publication of this book. I have no words to describe the role, efforts, inputs and initiatives undertaken by **Mr Bhupesh Aarora** [Sr. Vice President – Publishing & Marketing (Health Sciences Division)] for helping and motivating me.

I sincerely thank the entire CBS team for bringing out the book with utmost care and attractive presentation. I would like to thank Ms Nitasha Arora (Assistant General Manager Publishing – Medical and Nursing), and Dr Anju Dhir (Sr. Product Manager and Medical Development Editor) for their publishing support. I would also extend my thanks to Ms Surbhi Gupta (Sr. English Editor), Mr Ashutosh Pathak (Sr. Proofreader cum Team Coordinator) and all the production team members for devoting laborious hours in designing and typesetting the book.

I am extremely thankful to my colleague Ms Simranjeet Kaur, faculty, Institute of Nursing Education, Guru Teg Bahadur Sahib (C) Hospital, Ludhiana, Punjab for providing encouragement and sound advice. I am also thankful to my parents for their constant guidance and motivation. They are always my never-ending source of support and inspiration.

# From the Publisher's Desk

*Dear Reader,*

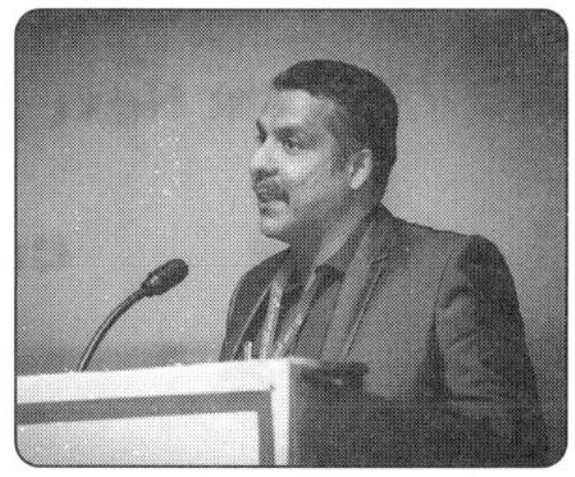

Nursing Education has a rich history, often characterized by traditional teaching techniques that have evolved over time. Primarily, teaching took place within classroom settings. Lectures, textbooks, and clinical rotations were the core teaching tools; and students majorly relied on textbooks by local or foreign publishers for quality education. However, today, technology has completely transformed the field of nursing education, making it an integral part of the curriculum. It has evolved to include a range of technological tools that enhance the learning experience and better prepare students for clinical practice.

As publishers, we've been contributing to the field of Medical Science, Nursing and Allied Sciences and earned the trust of many. By supporting **Indian authors**, coupled with **nursing webinars and conferences**, we have paved an easier path for aspiring nurses, empowering them to excel in national and state level exams. With this, we're not only enhancing the quality of patient care but also enabling future nurses to adapt to new challenges and innovations in the rapidly evolving world of healthcare. Following the ideology of **Bringing learning to people instead of people going for learning**, so far, we've been doing our part by:

- Developing quality content by qualified and well-versed authors
- Building a strong community of faculty and students
- Introducing a smart approach with Digital/Hybrid Books, and
- Offering simulation Nursing Procedures, etc.

Innovative teaching methodologies, such as modern-age Phygital Books, have sparked the interest of the Next-Gen students in pursuing advanced education. The enhancement of educational standards through **Omnipresent Knowledge Sharing Platforms** has further facilitated learning, bridging the gap between doctors and nurses.

At Nursing Next Live, a sister concern of CBS Publishers & Distributors, we have long recognized the immense potential within the nursing field. Our journey in innovating nursing education has allowed us to make substantial and meaningful contributions. With the vision of strengthening learning at every stage, we have introduced several plans that cater to the specific needs of the students, including but not limited to **Plan UG** for undergraduates, **Plan MSc** for postgraduate aspirants, **Plan FDP** for upskilling faculties, **SDL** for integrated learning and **Plan NP** for bridging the gap between theoretical & practical learning. Additionally, we have successfully completed seven series of our **Target High** Book in a very short period, setting a milestone in the education industry. We have been able to achieve all this just with the sole vision of laying the foundation of diversified knowledge for all. With the rise of a new generation of educated, tech-savvy individuals, we anticipate even more remarkable advancements in the coming years.

We take immense pride in our achievements and eagerly look forward to the future, brimming with new opportunities for innovation, growth and collaborations with experienced minds such as yourself who can contribute to our mission as Authors, Reviewers and/or Faculties. Together, let's foster a generation of nurses who are confident, competent, and prepared to succeed in a technology-driven healthcare system.

**Mr Bhupesh Aarora**
(Sr Vice President – Publishing & Marketing)
bhupeshaarora@cbspd.com| +91 95553 53330

# Contents

*Preface* ........ *v*
*Acknowledgments* ........ *vii*

## Nursing Health History

- Nursing Health History–1 ........ 32
- Nursing Health History–2 ........ 39

## General Physical Examination

- General Physical Examination–1 ........ 46
- General Physical Examination–2 ........ 58

## Nursing Care Plan

- Nursing Care Plan–1 ........ 70
- Nursing Care Plan–2 ........ 100
- Nursing Care Plan–3 ........ 130
- Nursing Care Plan–4 ........ 160

## Health Education

- Health Education ........ 188

# *Student's Identification Profile*

Paste Your
Passport
Size Photograph

**Name of the Student:** ________________________________

**Registration No./Enrolment No.:** ________________________________

**Course/Year:** ________________________________

**Subject:** ________________________________

**Batch:** ________________________________

**University:** ________________________________

**Name of the Institute:** ________________________________

**Address of the Institute:** ________________________________

: ________________________________

: ________________________________

: ________________________________

| ________________ | ________________ | ________________ |
|---|---|---|
| **Signature of the Student** | **Signature of the Subject Coordinator/HOD** | **Signature of the Principal** |

## EVALUATION

| Sl. No. | Content | Marks Obtained | Maximum Marks |
|---|---|---|---|
| I. | Health Education | | 25 |
| II. | Observation Report of CSSD | | 25 |
| III. | Nursing Health History | | |
| | 1. | | 10 |
| | 2. | | 10 |
| IV. | General Physical Examination | | |
| | 1. | | 15 |
| | 2. | | 15 |
| V. | Nursing Care Plan | | |
| | 1. | | 25 |
| | 2. | | 25 |
| | 3. | | 25 |
| | 4. | | 25 |

# Nursing Foundations-I (Semester I)

## Syllabus for BSc (Nursing) Semester I
## Nursing Foundations-I (Including First Aid Module)
## Practical

**Placement:** Semester I

**Time:** Practicum: Skill Lab: 2 Credits (80 hours) and Clinical: 2 Credits (160 hours)

| Clinical unit | Duration (in weeks) | Learning outcomes | Procedural competencies/ clinical skills (supervised clinical practice) | Clinical requirements | Assessment methods |
|---|---|---|---|---|---|
| General Medical/ Surgical Wards | 2 | • Maintain effective human relations (projecting professional image)<br>• Communicate effectively with patient, families and team members<br>• Demonstrate skills in techniques of recording and reporting | **Communication and Nurse Patient Relationship**<br>• Maintaining communication with patient and family and interpersonal relationship<br>• Documentation and reporting<br>▪ Documenting patient care and procedures<br>▪ Verbal report<br>▪ Written report | | • OSCE |
| | 2 | • Demonstrate skill in monitoring vital signs<br>• Care for patients with altered vital signs<br>• Demonstrate skill in implementing standard precautions and use of PPE | **Vital Signs**<br>• Monitor/measure and document vital signs in a graphic sheet<br>▪ Temperature (oral, tympanic, axillary)<br>▪ Pulse (apical and peripheral pulses)<br>▪ Respiration<br>▪ Blood pressure<br>▪ Pulse oximetry<br>• Interpret and report alteration<br>• Cold applications – cold compress, ice cap, tepid sponging<br>• Care of equipment – thermometer, BP apparatus, stethoscope, pulse oximeter<br>*Infection Control in Clinical Settings*<br>• Hand hygiene<br>• Use of PPE | • Care of patients with alterations in vital signs | • Assessment of clinical skills using checklist<br>• OSCE |

| Clinical unit | Duration (in weeks) | Learning outcomes | Procedural competencies/ clinical skills (supervised clinical practice) | Clinical requirements | Assessment methods |
|---|---|---|---|---|---|
| | 3 | • Demonstrate skill in meeting the comfort needs of the patients<br><br>• Provide safe and clean environment | **Comfort, Rest & Sleep, Pain and Promoting Safety in Health Care Environment**<br>*Comfort, Rest & Sleep*<br>• Bed making:<br>▪ Open<br>▪ Closed<br>▪ Occupied<br>▪ Postoperative<br>▪ Cardiac bed<br>▪ Fracture bed<br>• Comfort devices<br>▪ Pillows<br>▪ Over bed table/ cardiac table<br>▪ Back rest<br>▪ Bed cradle<br>• Therapeutic positions<br>▪ Supine<br>▪ Fowler's (low, semi, high)<br>▪ Lateral<br>▪ Prone<br>▪ Sim's<br>▪ Trendelenburg<br>▪ Dorsal recumbent<br>▪ Lithotomy<br>▪ Knee chest<br>*Pain*<br>• Pain assessment and provision for comfort<br>*Promoting Safety in Health Care Environment*<br>• Care of patient's unit<br>• Use of safety devices:<br>▪ Side rails<br>• Restraints (physical)<br>• Fall risk assessment and post fall assessment | • Fall risk assessment-1 | • Assessment of clinical skills using checklist<br>• OSCE |

| Clinical unit | Duration (in weeks) | Learning outcomes | Procedural competencies/ clinical skills (supervised clinical practice) | Clinical requirements | Assessment methods |
|---|---|---|---|---|---|
| | 2 | Demonstrate skill in admission, transfer, and discharge of a patient | **Hospital Admission and Discharge, Mobility and Immobility and Patient education**<br>*Hospital Admission and Discharge*<br>Perform & document:<br>• Admission<br>• Transfer<br>• Planned discharge | | • Assessment of clinical skills using checklist<br>• OSCE |
| | | • Demonstrate skill in caring for patients with restricted mobility<br>• Plan and provide appropriate health teaching following the principles | *Mobility and Immobility*<br>• Range of motion exercises<br>• Assist patient in:<br>  ▪ Moving<br>  ▪ Turning<br>  ▪ Logrolling<br>• Changing position of helpless patient<br>• Transferring (Bed to and from chair/ wheelchair/stretcher)<br>*Patient Education* | • Individual teaching-1 | • Assessment of clinical skills using checklist<br>• OSCE |
| | 1 | Demonstrate skills in assessing and performing first aid during emergencies | **First Aid and Emergencies**<br>• Bandaging techniques<br>  ▪ Basic bandages:<br>    ◊ Circular<br>    ◊ Spiral<br>    ◊ Reverse-spiral<br>    ◊ Recurrent<br>    ◊ Figure of eight<br>  ▪ Special bandages:<br>    ◊ Caplin<br>    ◊ Eye/ear bandage<br>    ◊ Jaw bandage<br>    ◊ Shoulder spica<br>    ◊ Thumb spica<br>    ◊ Triangular bandage/sling (head & limbs)<br>    ◊ Binders | • Module completion<br>• National Disaster Management Authority (NDMA) First Aid module (to complete it in clinicals if not completed during lab) | • Assessment of clinical skills using checklist<br>• OSCE (first aid compe- tencies) |

## SEMESTER I

| Sl. No. | Competencies | Demonstration | | Return Demonstration | |
|---|---|---|---|---|---|
| | | Date | Signature | Date | Signature |
| 1 | Therapeutic communication and documentation | | | | |
| 2 | Vital signs | | | | |
| 3 | Medical and surgical asepsis | | | | |
| 4 | Pain assessment | | | | |
| 5 | Comfort devices | | | | |
| 6 | Therapeutic positions | | | | |
| 7 | Physical restraints and side rails | | | | |
| 8 | ROM exercises | | | | |
| 9 | Ambulation | | | | |
| 10 | Moving and turning patients in bed | | | | |
| 11 | Changing position of helpless patients | | | | |
| 12 | Transferring patients bed to stretcher/wheelchair | | | | |
| 13 | Admission, transfer, discharge & health teaching | | | | |

## EVALUATION CRITERIA FOR HEALTH EDUCATION

Name of the Student: ______________________

Topic: ______________________ Area/Venue: ______________________

Date: ______________________ Time & Duration: ______________________

Group: ______________________

Name of the Supervisor: ______________________

| Sl. No. | Evaluation Criteria | Marks Obtained | Maximum Marks |
|---|---|---|---|
| 1 | Communication skills | | 2 |
| 2 | Objectives | | 1 |
| 3 | Content | | 3 |
| 4 | Preparation and effective use of AV aids | | 2 |
| 5 | Effectiveness of presentation | | 3 |
| 6 | Group participation | | 1 |
| 7 | Time management | | 1 |
| 8 | Bibliography | | 1 |
| 9 | Timely submission | | 1 |
| **Total marks** | | | **15** |

**Remarks:** ______________________

______________________

______________________

______________________

______________________

**Signature of the Student** **Signature of the Clinical Supervisor**

**Date:** ______________________ **Date:** ______________________

# HEALTH EDUCATION

Name of the Student: ____________________

Topic: ____________________ Area/Venue: ____________________

Date: ____________________ Time & Duration: ____________________

Group: ____________________

Name of the Supervisor: ____________________

## OBJECTIVES

At the end of the teaching, the group will be able to:

## GENERAL OBJECTIVE

## SPECIFIC OBJECTIVES

## LESSON PLAN

| Specific objectives | Time & duration | Content | Teaching-learning activities | AV aids used |
|---|---|---|---|---|
| | | | | |

| Specific objectives | Time & duration | Content | Teaching-learning activities | AV aids used |
|---|---|---|---|---|
| | | | | |

| Specific objectives | Time & duration | Content | Teaching-learning activities | AV aids used |
|---|---|---|---|---|
| | | | | |

| Specific objectives | Time & duration | Content | Teaching-learning activities | AV aids used |
|---|---|---|---|---|
| | | | | |

| Specific objectives | Time & duration | Content | Teaching-learning activities | AV aids used |
|---|---|---|---|---|
| | | | | |

## BIBLIOGRAPHY

## EVALUATION CRITERIA FOR OBSERVATION REPORT

Name of the Student: ____________________

Area of Observation: ____________________ Date of Visit: ____________________

Name of the Supervisor: ____________________

| Sl. No. | Evaluation Criteria | Marks Obtained | Maximum Marks |
|---|---|---|---|
| 1 | Objectives | | 2 |
| 2 | Physical setup of CSSD | | 3 |
| 3 | Staffing pattern of CSSD | | 3 |
| 4 | Functions of CSSD | | 2 |
| 5 | Major areas/divisions in CSSD | | 2 |
| 6 | Sterilization and disinfection facilities | | 2 |
| 7 | Timely submission | | 1 |
| **Total marks** | | | **15** |

**Remarks:** ____________________

____________________

____________________

____________________

____________________

**Signature of the Student**

**Date:** ____________________

**Signature of the Clinical Supervisor**

**Date:** ____________________

# OBSERVATION REPORT OF CENTRAL STERILE SERVICES DEPARTMENT (CSSD)

Date of Visit: ____________________

**Objectives**

**Introduction to CSSD**

**Physical Setup of CSSD**

**Staffing Pattern of CSSD**

**Functions of CSSD**

**Major Areas/Divisions in CSSD**

**Sterilization and Disinfection Facilities**

# Nursing Foundations-II
# (Semester II)

## Syllabus for BSc (Nursing) Semester II
## Nursing Foundations-II (Including Health Assessment Module)
## Practical

**Placement:** Semester II
**Time:** Practicum: Skill Lab: 3 Credits 120 hours) and Clinical: 4 Credits (320 hours)

| Clinical unit | Duration (in weeks) | Learning outcomes | Procedural competencies/clinical skills (supervised clinical practice) | Clinical requirements | Assessment methods |
|---|---|---|---|---|---|
| General Medical/ Surgical Wards | 3 | Perform health assessment of each body system | **Health Assessment**<br>• Nursing/health history taking<br>• Perform physical examination:<br>▪ General<br>▪ Body systems<br>• Use various methods of physical examination—inspection, palpation, percussion, auscultation, olfaction<br>• Identification of system-wise deviations<br>• Documentation of findings | • History taking – 2<br>• Physical examination – 2 | • Assessment of clinical skills using checklist<br>• OSCE |
| | 1 | Develop skills in assessment, planning, implementation and evaluation of nursing care using nursing process approach | **The Nursing Process**<br>• Prepare nursing care plan for the patient based on the given case scenario | • Nursing process – 1 | • Evaluation of nursing process with criteria |
| | 2 | Identify and meet the nutritional needs of patients | **Nutritional Needs, Elimination Needs & Diagnostic Testing**<br>*Nutritional Needs*<br>• Nutritional assessment<br>• Preparation of nasogastric tube feed<br>• Nasogastric tube feeding | • Nutritional assessment and clinical presentation – 1 | • Assessment of clinical skills using checklist<br>• OSCE |

| Clinical unit | Duration (in weeks) | Learning outcomes | Procedural competencies/clinical skills (supervised clinical practice) | Clinical requirements | Assessment methods |
|---|---|---|---|---|---|
| | | Implement basic nursing techniques in meeting hygienic needs of patients | *Hygiene*<br>• Care of skin & hair:<br>▪ Sponge bath/bed bath<br>▪ Care of pressure points & back massage<br>• Pressure sore risk assessment using Braden/Norton scale<br>▪ Hair wash<br>▪ Pediculosis treatment<br>• Oral hygiene<br>• Perineal hygiene<br>• Catheter care | • Pressure sore assessment – 1 | |
| | 2 | • Plan and implement care to meet the elimination needs of patient<br>• Develop skills in instructing and collecting samples for investigation<br>• Perform simple lab tests and analyze & interpret common diagnostic values | **Elimination Needs**<br>• Providing<br>▪ Urinal<br>▪ Bedpan<br>• Insertion of Suppository<br>• Enema<br>• Urinary catheter care<br>• Care of urinary drainage<br>**Diagnostic testing**<br>• Specimen collection<br>▪ Urine routine and culture<br>▪ Stool routine<br>▪ Sputum culture<br>• Perform simple lab tests using reagent strips<br>▪ Urine – glucose, albumin, acetone, pH, specific gravity<br>• Blood – GRBS monitoring | • Clinical presentation on care of patient with constipation – 1<br>• Lab values – interpretation | • Assessment of clinical skills using checklist<br>• OSCE |

| Clinical unit | Duration (in weeks) | Learning outcomes | Procedural competencies/clinical skills (supervised clinical practice) | Clinical requirements | Assessment methods |
|---|---|---|---|---|---|
| | 3 | • Identify patients with impaired oxygenation and demonstrate skill in caring for patients with impaired oxygenation<br><br>• Identify and demonstrate skill in caring for patients with fluid, electrolyte and acid – base imbalances | **Oxygenation Needs, Fluid, Electrolyte, and Acid-Base Balances**<br>***Oxygenation Needs***<br>• Oxygen administration methods<br>▪ Nasal prongs<br>▪ Face mask/venturi mask<br>• Steam inhalation<br>• Chest physiotherapy<br>• Deep breathing & coughing exercises<br>• Oral suctioning<br>***Fluid, Electrolyte, and Acid-Base Balances***<br>• Maintaining intake output chart<br>• Identify & report complications of IV therapy<br>• Observe blood & blood component therapy<br>• Identify & report complications of blood & blood component therapy | | • Assessment of clinical skills using checklist<br>• OSCE<br>• Assessment of clinical skills using checklist<br>• OSCE |

| Clinical unit | Duration (in weeks) | Learning outcomes | Procedural competencies/clinical skills (supervised clinical practice) | Clinical requirements | Assessment methods |
|---|---|---|---|---|---|
| | 3 | • Explain the principles, routes, effects of administration of medications<br>• Calculate conversions of drugs and dosages within and between systems of measurements<br>• Administer drugs by the following routes—oral, intradermal, subcutaneous, intramuscular, intravenous topical, inhalation | **Administration of Medications**<br>• Calculate drug dosages<br>• Preparation of lotions & solutions<br>• Administer medications<br>▪ Oral<br>▪ Topical<br>▪ Inhalations<br>▪ Parenteral<br>◊ Intradermal<br>◊ Subcutaneous<br>◊ Intramuscular<br>◊ Instillations<br>▪ Eye, ear, nose—instillation of medicated drops, nasal sprays, irrigations | | • Assessment of clinical skills using checklist<br>• OSCE |
| | 2 | • Assess, plan, implement & evaluate the basic care needs of patients with altered functioning of sense organs and unconsciousness<br>• Care for terminally ill and dying patients | **Sensory Needs and Care of Unconscious Patients, Care of Terminally Ill, Death and Dying**<br>*Sensory Needs and Care of Unconscious Patients*<br>• Assessment of level of consciousness using Glasgow Coma Scale<br>*Terminally Ill, Death and Dying*<br>• Death care | • Nursing rounds on care of patient with altered sensorium | • Assessment of clinical skills using checklist<br>• OSCE<br>• Assessment of clinical skills using checklist |

## SEMESTER II

| Sl. No. | Competencies | Demonstration | | Return Demonstration | |
|---|---|---|---|---|---|
| | | Date | Signature | Date | Signature |
| 1 | Health assessment | | | | |
| 2 | Nutritional assessment | | | | |
| 3 | • Sponge bath<br>• Oral hygiene<br>• Perineal care | | | | |
| 4 | Nasogastric tube feeding | | | | |
| 5 | Providing bedpan & urinal | | | | |
| 6 | Catheter care | | | | |
| 7 | • Bowel wash<br>• Enema<br>• Insertion of suppository | | | | |
| 8 | Oxygen administration—<br>• Face mask<br>• Venturi mask<br>• Nasal prongs | | | | |
| 9 | Administration of medication through parenteral route—<br>• IM<br>• SC<br>• ID<br>• IV | | | | |
| 10 | Last office | | | | |

# EVALUATION CRITERIA FOR NURSING HEALTH HISTORY

Name of the Student: ______________________________

Diagnosis of Patient: ______________________________

Ward/Unit: ____________________ Date of Submission: ____________________

<table>
<tr><th>Sl. No.</th><th>Evaluation Criteria</th><th>Marks Obtained</th><th colspan="2">Maximum Marks</th></tr>
<tr><td>1.</td><td>Utilized therapeutic communication skills while interacting with patient and his/her family members</td><td></td><td colspan="2">2</td></tr>
<tr><td>2.</td><td>Collected thorough and accurate patient information:<br>• Biographical data of the patient<br>• Chief complaints<br>• History of present illness<br>• Past health history<br>• Family history<br>• Lifestyle<br>• Environmental history</td><td></td><td>1<br>1<br>1<br>1<br>1<br>1<br>1</td><td>7</td></tr>
<tr><td>3.</td><td>Timely submission</td><td></td><td colspan="2">1</td></tr>
<tr><td colspan="2">Total marks</td><td></td><td colspan="2">10</td></tr>
</table>

**Remarks:** ______________________________

______________________________

______________________________

**Signature of the Student**

**Signature of the Clinical Supervisor**

**Date:** ____________

**Date:** ____________

# NURSING HEALTH HISTORY–1

Date of collection of health history: ________ / ________ / ________

## I. BIOGRAPHICAL DATA OF THE PATIENT

Name of the patient: ______________________________

Father/Husband's name: ______________________________

Age: ______________ Gender: Male/Female ______________

Hospital: ______________________________

C.R./IP No.: ____________ Ward: ____________ Bed No.: ____________

Educational status: ______________ Occupation: ______________

Religion: ______________ Marital status: ______________

Address: ______________________________

______________________________

Date of admission: ______________________________

Treatment under Dr.: ______________________________

Diagnosis: ______________________________

Surgery performed, if any: ______________________________

Date of surgery performed: ______________________________

## II. CHIEF COMPLAINTS

At the time of admission: ________________________________

At present:

## III. HISTORY OF PRESENT ILLNESS

(Includes details about chief complaints: Character, onset-sudden/gradual, location, duration, severity, pattern, aggravating factors, relieving factors, associated manifestations)

## IV. PAST HEALTH HISTORY

(a) Childhood illness: ________________________________

________________________________

(b) Adult illnesses: ________________________________

________________________________

(c) Psychiatric illnesses: ________________________________

________________________________

(d) Previous hospitalizations: ________________________________

________________________________

________________________________

(e) Previous surgical or diagnostic procedures: ________________________________

________________________________

(f) Allergies to foods/medications: ________________________________

________________________________

(g) Menstrual history (for female patient):

Last menstrual period (LMP): ________________ Menopausal: Yes/No ________________

Age at menarche: ____________ years. Menstruation: Regular/irregular duration: ____________

Does bleeding/spotting occur between periods: Yes/No ________________

Is pain associated with periods: ________________________________

(h) Past obstetrical history:

Have never been pregnant: ________________________________

Birth control/contraception: ________________________________

| **Number of pregnancies** | **Year** | **Pregnancy** (normal/miscarriage/abortion) | **Delivery** (normal/assisted/ cesarean section) | **Gender of baby** | **Puerperium** (normal/ complicated) |
|---|---|---|---|---|---|
| | | | | | |
| | | | | | |
| | | | | | |
| | | | | | |
| | | | | | |
| | | | | | |
| | | | | | |
| | | | | | |
| | | | | | |
| | | | | | |

## V. FAMILY HISTORY

(a) Family composition:

| Name | Age | Gender | Relationship with patient | Educational status | Occupation | Income | Health status |
|---|---|---|---|---|---|---|---|
| | | | | | | | |

(b) Family tree/genogram:

Key:

Male

Female

Patient

Deceased

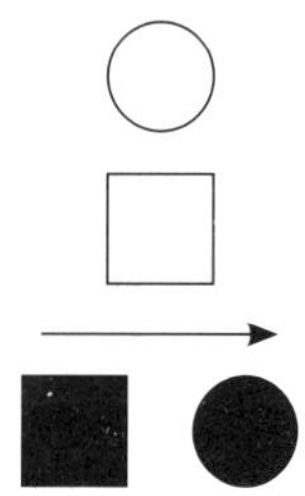

(c) History of any recent death in family: Yes/No

Relationship with patient: ______________________ Age at death: ______________________

Cause of death: ______________________________________________

(d) History of any chronic illness in family:

(Hypertension, heart disease, diabetes, tuberculosis, asthma, renal disorder, arthritis, cancer, allergies, epilepsy, mental illness, etc.): Yes/No

If yes, give details: ______________________________________________

______________________________________________

______________________________________________

(e) History of any communicable disease in family: ____________________

____________________

____________________

(f) History of any hereditary disease in family: ____________________

____________________

____________________

## VI. LIFESTYLE

(a) Diet: Vegetarian/eggetarian/nonvegetarian/special diet: ____________________

____________________

(b) Bowel and bladder habit: ____________________

____________________

(c) Use of any addictive or illicit substance/drug (heroine/cocaine/alcohol/tobacco): Yes/No

____________________

____________________

____________________

____________________

(d) Sleeping pattern: ____________________

____________________

(e) Exercise: ____________________

____________________

(f) Recreation: ____________________

____________________

(g) Religious belief: ____________________

____________________

## VII. ENVIRONMENTAL HISTORY

(a) Physical-type of housing: ________________________________________________

________________________________________________

(b) Environmental hygiene: ________________________________________________

________________________________________________

(c) Source of drinking water: ________________________________________________

________________________________________________

(d) Presence of flies/mosquitoes/rodents: ________________________________________________

________________________________________________

(e) Disposal of excreta: ________________________________________________

________________________________________________

(f) Environmental pollution: ________________________________________________

________________________________________________

(g) Exposure to hazardous waste: ________________________________________________

________________________________________________

## EVALUATION CRITERIA FOR NURSING HEALTH HISTORY

Name of the Student: ______________________________

Diagnosis of Patient: ______________________________

Ward/Unit: ____________________ Date of Submission: ____________________

<table>
<tr><th>Sl. No.</th><th>Evaluation Criteria</th><th>Marks Obtained</th><th colspan="2">Maximum Marks</th></tr>
<tr><td>1.</td><td>Utilized therapeutic communication skills while interacting with patient and his/her family members</td><td></td><td colspan="2">2</td></tr>
<tr><td>2.</td><td>Collected thorough and accurate patient information:<br>• Biographical data of the patient<br>• Chief complaints<br>• History of present illness<br>• Past health history<br>• Family history<br>• Lifestyle<br>• Environmental history</td><td></td><td><br>1<br>1<br>1<br>1<br>1<br>1<br>1</td><td>7</td></tr>
<tr><td>3.</td><td>Timely submission</td><td></td><td colspan="2">1</td></tr>
<tr><td colspan="2">Total marks</td><td></td><td colspan="2">10</td></tr>
</table>

**Remarks:** ______________________________

______________________________

______________________________

______________________ ______________________

**Signature of the Student** **Signature of the Clinical Supervisor**

**Date:** ____________ **Date:** ____________

# NURSING HEALTH HISTORY–2

Date of collection of health history: ________ / ________ / ________

## I. BIOGRAPHICAL DATA OF THE PATIENT

Name of the patient: ______________________________

Father/Husband's name: ______________________________

Age: ______________ Gender: Male/Female ______________

Hospital: ______________________________

C.R./IP No.: __________ Ward: __________ Bed No.: __________

Educational status: ______________ Occupation: ______________

Religion: ______________ Marital status: ______________

Address: ______________________________

______________________________

Date of admission: ______________________________

Treatment under Dr.: ______________________________

Diagnosis: ______________________________

Surgery performed, if any: ______________________________

Date of surgery performed: ______________________________

## II. CHIEF COMPLAINTS

At the time of admission: ______________________________

______________________________

______________________________

______________________________

At present:

______________________________

______________________________

______________________________

______________________________

______________________________

______________________________

## III. HISTORY OF PRESENT ILLNESS

(Includes details about chief complaints: Character, onset-sudden/gradual, location, duration, severity, pattern, aggravating factors, relieving factors, associated manifestations)

______________________________

______________________________

______________________________

______________________________

______________________________

______________________________

______________________________

______________________________

______________________________

______________________________

______________________________

## IV. PAST HEALTH HISTORY

(a) Childhood illness: ______________________________

______________________________

(b) Adult illnesses: ______________________________

______________________________

(c) Psychiatric illnesses: ______________________________

______________________________

(d) Previous hospitalizations: ______________________________

______________________________

______________________________

(e) Previous surgical or diagnostic procedures: ______________________________

______________________________

(f) Allergies to foods/medications: ______________________________

______________________________

(g) Menstrual history (for female patient):

Last menstrual period (LMP): ______________ Menopausal: Yes/No ______________

Age at menarche: ______________ years. Menstruation: Regular/irregular duration: ______________

Does bleeding/spotting occur between periods: Yes/No ______________

Is pain associated with periods: ______________

(h) Past obstetrical history:

Have never been pregnant: ______________

Birth control/contraception: ______________

| Number of pregnancies | Year | Pregnancy (normal/miscarriage/abortion) | Delivery (normal/assisted/ cesarean section) | Gender of baby | Puerperium (normal/ complicated) |
|---|---|---|---|---|---|
| | | | | | |
| | | | | | |
| | | | | | |
| | | | | | |
| | | | | | |
| | | | | | |
| | | | | | |
| | | | | | |
| | | | | | |
| | | | | | |

## V. FAMILY HISTORY

(a) Family composition:

| Name | Age | Gender | Relationship with patient | Educational status | Occupation | Income | Health status |
|---|---|---|---|---|---|---|---|
| | | | | | | | |

(b) Family tree/genogram:

Key:

Male

Female

Patient

Deceased

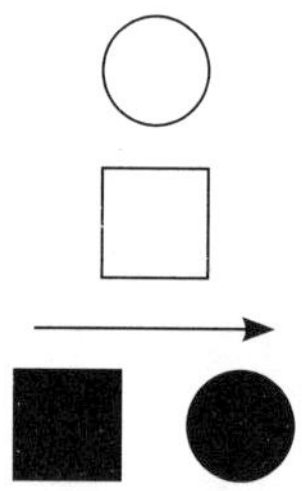

(c) History of any recent death in family: Yes/No

Relationship with patient: ______________________ Age at death: ______________________

Cause of death: ______________________________________________

(d) History of any chronic illness in family:

(Hypertension, heart disease, diabetes, tuberculosis, asthma, renal disorder, arthritis, cancer, allergies, epilepsy, mental illness, etc.): Yes/No

If yes, give details: ______________________________________________

______________________________________________

______________________________________________

(e) History of any communicable disease in family: ______________________________

______________________________

______________________________

(f) History of any hereditary disease in family: ______________________________

______________________________

______________________________

## VI. LIFESTYLE

(a) Diet: Vegetarian/eggetarian/nonvegetarian/special diet: ______________________________

______________________________

(b) Bowel and bladder habit: ______________________________

______________________________

(c) Use of any addictive or illicit substance/drug (heroine/cocaine/alcohol/tobacco): Yes/No

______________________________

______________________________

______________________________

______________________________

(d) Sleeping pattern: ______________________________

______________________________

(e) Exercise: ______________________________

______________________________

(f) Recreation: ______________________________

______________________________

(g) Religious belief: ______________________________

______________________________

## VII. ENVIRONMENTAL HISTORY

(a) Physical-type of housing: ______________________________

______________________________

(b) Environmental hygiene: ______________________________

______________________________

(c) Source of drinking water: ______________________________

______________________________

(d) Presence of flies/mosquitoes/rodents: ______________________________

______________________________

(e) Disposal of excreta: ______________________________

______________________________

(f) Environmental pollution: ______________________________

______________________________

(g) Exposure to hazardous waste: ______________________________

______________________________

## EVALUATION CRITERIA FOR GENERAL PHYSICAL EXAMINATION

Name of the Student: ______________________________

Clinical Diagnosis of Patient: ______________________________

Ward/Unit: ____________________ Date of Performing GPE: ____________________

| Sl. No. | Evaluation Criteria | Marks Obtained | Maximum Marks |
|---|---|---|---|
| 1 | Utilized therapeutic communication skills while interacting with patient | | 2 |
| 2 | Subjective assessment | | 5 |
| 3 | Objective assessment | | 5 |
| 4 | Use of fundamental techniques (inspection, palpation, percussion and auscultation) | | 2 |
| 5 | Timely submission | | 1 |
| | **Total marks** | | **15** |

**Remarks:** ______________________________

______________________________

______________________________

______________________________

**Signature of the Student**

**Signature of the Clinical Supervisor**

**Date:** ____________________

**Date:** ____________________

# GENERAL PHYSICAL EXAMINATION–1

## I. GENERAL APPEARANCE

Level of consciousness (conscious/semiconscious/unconscious/coma): ____________________

Orientation (time, place and person): ____________________

____________________

____________________

Activity (active/dull): ____________________

Body built (average/thin/obese): ____________________

Look (anxious/depressed): ____________________

Posture (Body curves: Lordosis/kyphosis/scoliosis): ____________________

## II. ANTHROPOMETRIC MEASUREMENT

Height: __________ Weight: __________ BMI: __________

[Body mass index; BMI = Weight (in kilograms)/Height$^2$ (in meters)]

## III. VITAL SIGNS

| Date/vitals | Temperature (in C°/F°) | Pulse (beats/min) | Respiration (breaths/min) | Blood pressure (in mm Hg) |
|---|---|---|---|---|
| | | | | |
| | | | | |
| | | | | |
| | | | | |
| | | | | |
| | | | | |
| | | | | |

| Area/subjective data | Objective data |
|---|---|
| **Head and Neck** | **Scalp:**<br>• Cleanliness: ______<br>• Abrasions/wound: ______<br>______<br>**Hairs:**<br>• Color: ______<br>• Texture (fine/coarse/brittle/dull): ______<br>• Distribution (hair loss): ______<br>• Dandruff: ______<br>• Pediculi or any other infection: ______<br>**Face (pale, puffiness, expressions, enlargement of parotid glands):** ______<br>______<br>**Neck:**<br>• Lump or mass: ______<br>• Lymphadenopathy: ______<br>• Range of motion (flexion, extension, rotation):<br>______<br>______<br>• Jugular venous pulses: ______<br>**Thyroid gland (landmarks, lump):**<br>______<br>______ |

*Contd...*

| Area/subjective data | Objective data |
|---|---|
| **Eyes** | **Eyelids:**<br>• Position (ptosis/lid retraction): ____________<br>**Lid margin:**<br>• Edema: ____________<br>• Erythema: ____________<br>• Lesions: ____________<br>**Sclera:**<br>____________<br>____________<br>**Conjunctiva:**<br>____________<br>____________<br>**Pupils:**<br>• Color: ____________<br>• Pupillary response: ____________<br>____________<br>____________<br>**Extraocular movements:**<br>____________<br>____________<br>Use of spectacles/contact lens: ____________<br>____________<br>Visual acuity: ____________<br>____________ |

*Contd...*

| Area/subjective data | Objective data |
|---|---|
| **Ears** | **Use of hearing aids:** ____________<br><br>**Auricle (deformity, lesion, discharge, size, symmetry, angle of attachment to head):** ____________<br>____________<br>____________<br>____________<br><br>**Mastoid area (tenderness):** ____________<br>____________<br><br>**External auditory canal (discharge/cerumen/fluid/blood, nodule):** ____________<br>____________<br><br>**Tympanic membrane (color):** ____________<br><br>**Hearing acuity:** ____________<br>• Whisper test: ____________<br>• Weber test: ____________<br>• Rinne test: ____________ |

*Contd...*

| Area/subjective data | Objective data |
|---|---|
| **Nose and Sinuses** | **External nose:**<br>• Lesions: ______<br>• Asymmetry: ______<br>• Inflammation: ______<br>**Internal structures of nose:**<br>• Nasal mucosa (color/swelling/exudates/bleeding/polyps):<br>______<br>______<br>______<br>______<br>Nasal septum (central/deviated): ______<br>**Sinuses:**<br>• Frontal sinuses: ______<br>• Maxillary sinuses: ______ |
| **Mouth and Pharynx** | Lips (symmetry, color, dry/moist):<br>______<br>Buccal mucosa (color/consistency/lesion/mass):<br>______<br>Gums (color/lesions/swelling/bleeding/discharge):<br>______<br>Odor from the mouth: ______<br>Teeth (total number of teeth, color, tooth decay):<br>______<br>Tongue (symmetry/color/texture/moisture): ______<br>Hard and soft palate (color/lesion):<br>______<br>Uvula (position/color):<br>______<br>Tonsils (color/size/exudate):<br>______<br>Pharynx (color/lesion/exudate):<br>______ |

*Contd...*

| Area/subjective data | Objective data |
|---|---|
| **Thorax/Lungs** | **Is client on: Room air/oxygen/ventilator**<br>If on oxygen support:<br>• Flow rate: __________<br>• Mode: __________<br>Endotracheal tube: Present/absent: __________<br>**Thorax:**<br>• Shape and symmetry: __________<br>• Position of sternum: __________<br>• Use of accessory muscles: __________<br>• Intercostal space (retraction/bulging): __________<br>• Respiratory rate: __________ Rhythm: __________<br>**Dyspnea (shortness of breath):**<br>• On rest: __________<br>• On exertion: __________<br>• Orthopnea: __________<br>• With expiratory/inspiratory wheezing: __________<br>**Cough:**<br>• Character (dry/hacking/brassy/wheezing): __________<br>• Time (morning/night): __________<br>**Sputum:**<br>• Color (colorless/yellowish/rust color/bright red/black):<br>__________<br>• Odor: __________<br>**Chest pain:**<br>• Location (left/right side): __________<br>• Sharp/stabbing/intermittent/dull/aching/persistent: __________<br>• Duration: __________<br>**Wheezing:**<br>• Heard with/without stethoscope: __________<br>Hemoptysis: __________<br>Abnormal breath sounds (crackles/wheezing): __________<br>**Trachea (position, mass):**<br>__________<br>__________<br>__________ |

*Contd...*

| Area/subjective data | Objective data |
|---|---|
| **Heart** | Chest pain: __________<br>__________<br>• Referred pain (radiates to neck/arm/jaw/shoulders/hands/back/abdomen): __________<br>__________<br>Palpitations: __________<br>Heart sounds: __________<br>Murmurs: __________ |
| **Breast and Axilla** | **Breast:**<br>• Size and symmetry: __________<br>• Color: __________<br>• Venous pattern: __________<br>• Thickening/edema: __________<br>• Ulceration/rashes: __________<br>• Scar: __________<br>**Areola:**<br>• Color: __________<br>• Lesion: __________<br>**Nipple:**<br>• Discharge: __________<br>• Retraction: __________<br>• Lesion: __________<br>**Axilla:**<br>• Tenderness: __________<br>• Axillary lymph nodes: __________ |

*Contd...*

| Area/subjective data | Objective data |
|---|---|
| **Abdomen** | Abdominal girth: ______<br>Scars/lesions/rashes: ______<br>Symmetry: ______<br>Abdominal contour: ______<br>Vomiting: ______<br>______<br>______<br>**Changes in bowel habits and stool characteristics:** ______<br>• Diarrhea: ______<br>• Constipation: ______<br>**Bowel sounds (normal/hypoactive/hyperactive/absent):** ______<br>______<br>**Tympany or dullness (during percussion):** ______<br>______<br>______<br>Ascites: ______<br>**Tenderness or swelling:**<br>• All quadrants: ______<br>• Liver: ______<br>• Spleen: ______<br>• Appendix: ______<br>• Kidney: ______<br>• Urinary bladder: ______ |

*Contd...*

| Area/subjective data | Objective data |
|---|---|
| **Genitalia** | Urinary catheter: Present/absent: ______<br>Urination (frequency, amount, color): ______<br>Urinary pattern (urgency, retention): ______<br>Burning micturition: ______<br>Hematuria: ______<br>**Male genitalia:**<br>• Penis: ______<br>• Scrotum: ______<br>• Inguinal area: ______<br>**Female genitalia:**<br>• Mons pubis: ______<br>• Labia majora: ______<br>• Urethra: ______<br>• Vagina: ______<br>• Cervix: ______ |
| **Anus and Rectum** | **Anus:**<br>• Anal opening area (redness, rashes, lump, ulcer, lesion, fissure, hemorrhoids): ______<br>______<br>Rectum (tenderness, smoothness, nodules): ______<br>______ |

*Contd...*

| Area/subjective data | Objective data |
|---|---|
| **Extremities** | Immobility: ______<br>Coordination: ______<br>Symmetry: ______<br>Capillary refill time: ______<br>Nails (cleanliness, color, clubbing, cyanosis): ______<br>______<br>______<br>Edema: ______<br>**Range of motion:**<br>• **Shoulder and arm:**<br>Flexion and hyperextension: ______<br>Adduction and abduction: ______<br>External and internal rotation: ______<br>• **Elbows:**<br>Flexion and extension: ______<br>Supination and pronation: ______<br>External and internal rotation: ______<br>• **Wrist:**<br>Flexion and extension: ______<br>• **Hands and fingers:**<br>Abduction and adduction: ______<br>Flexion and hyperextension: ______<br>• **Hips:**<br>Abduction and adduction: ______<br>Flexion and hyperextension: ______<br>• **Knees:**<br>Flexion and hyperextension: ______<br>• **Ankles and feet:**<br>Dorsiflexion and plantar flexion: ______<br>Eversion and inversion: ______<br>Abduction and adduction: ______<br>Varicose veins: ______ |

*Contd...*

| Area/subjective data | Objective data |
|---|---|
| Skin | **Color changes:**<br>• Pallor: ____________________<br>• Jaundice: ____________________<br>• Cyanosis: ____________________<br>Temperature (warm/normal/cold and clammy): ____________________<br>____________________<br>Skin texture (rough/smooth): ____________________<br>Skin turgor: ____________________<br>Skin integrity (intact/bedsores): ____________________<br>____________________<br>Edema: ____________________<br>Rash (location, itching): ____________________<br>Lesions (macule/papule/vesicle/nodule/pustule/scar): ____________________<br>____________________ |

## EVALUATION CRITERIA FOR GENERAL PHYSICAL EXAMINATION

Name of the Student: ____________________

Clinical diagnosis of Patient: ____________________

Ward/Unit: ____________________ Date of Performing GPE: ____________________

| Sl. No. | Evaluation Criteria | Marks Obtained | Maximum Marks |
|---|---|---|---|
| 1 | Utilized therapeutic communication skills while interacting with patient | | 2 |
| 2 | Subjective assessment | | 5 |
| 3 | Objective assessment | | 5 |
| 4 | Use of fundamental techniques (inspection, palpation, percussion and auscultation) | | 2 |
| 5 | Timely submission | | 1 |
| | **Total marks** | | **15** |

**Remarks:** ____________________

____________________

____________________

____________________

**Signature of the Student**

**Date:** ____________________

**Signature of the Clinical Supervisor**

**Date:** ____________________

# GENERAL PHYSICAL EXAMINATION–2

## I. GENERAL APPEARANCE

Level of consciousness (conscious/semiconscious/unconscious/coma): ______________________

Orientation (time, place and person): ______________________

______________________

______________________

Activity (active/dull): ______________________

Body built (average/thin/obese): ______________________

Look (anxious/depressed): ______________________

Posture (Body curves: Lordosis/kyphosis/scoliosis): ______________________

## II. ANTHROPOMETRIC MEASUREMENT

Height: ______________ Weight: ______________ BMI: ______________

[Body mass index; BMI = Weight (in kilograms)/Height$^2$ (in meters)]

## III. VITAL SIGNS

| Date/vitals | Temperature (in C°/F°) | Pulse (beats/min) | Respiration (breaths/min) | Blood pressure (in mm Hg) |
|---|---|---|---|---|
| | | | | |
| | | | | |
| | | | | |
| | | | | |
| | | | | |
| | | | | |
| | | | | |

| Area/subjective data | Objective data |
|---|---|
| **Head and Neck** | **Scalp:**<br>• Cleanliness: __________<br>• Abrasions/wound: __________<br>__________<br>**Hairs:**<br>• Color: __________<br>• Texture (fine/coarse/brittle/dull): __________<br>• Distribution (hair loss): __________<br>• Dandruff: __________<br>• Pediculi or any other infection: __________<br>**Face (pale, puffiness, expressions, enlargement of parotid glands):** __________<br>__________<br>**Neck:**<br>• Lump or mass: __________<br>• Lymphadenopathy: __________<br>• Range of motion (flexion, extension, rotation):<br>__________<br>__________<br>• Jugular venous pulses: __________<br>**Thyroid gland (landmarks, lump):**<br>__________<br>__________ |

*Contd...*

<table>
<tr><th>Area/subjective data</th><th>Objective data</th></tr>
<tr><td>Eyes</td><td>Eyelids:<br>• Position (ptosis/lid retraction): ____<br>Lid margin:<br>• Edema: ____<br>• Erythema: ____<br>• Lesions: ____<br>Sclera:<br>____<br>____<br>Conjunctiva:<br>____<br>____<br>Pupils:<br>• Color: ____<br>• Pupillary response: ____<br>____<br>____<br>Extraocular movements:<br>____<br>____<br>Use of spectacles/contact lens: ____<br>____<br>Visual acuity: ____<br>____</td></tr>
</table>

*Contd...*

| Area/subjective data | Objective data |
|---|---|
| **Ears** | **Use of hearing aids:** ____________<br><br>**Auricle (deformity, lesion, discharge, size, symmetry, angle of attachment to head):** ____________<br>____________<br>____________<br>____________<br><br>**Mastoid area (tenderness):** ____________<br>____________<br><br>**External auditory canal (discharge/cerumen/fluid/blood, nodule):** ____________<br>____________<br><br>**Tympanic membrane (color):** ____________<br><br>**Hearing acuity:** ____________<br><br>• Whisper test: ____________<br><br>• Weber test: ____________<br><br>• Rinne test: ____________ |

*Contd...*

| Area/subjective data | Objective data |
|---|---|
| **Nose and Sinuses** | **External nose:**<br>• Lesions: ____________<br>• Asymmetry: ____________<br>• Inflammation: ____________<br>**Internal structures of nose:**<br>• Nasal mucosa (color/swelling/exudates/bleeding/polyps):<br>____________<br>____________<br>____________<br>____________<br>Nasal septum (central/deviated): ____________<br>**Sinuses:**<br>• Frontal sinuses: ____________<br>• Maxillary sinuses: ____________ |
| **Mouth and Pharynx** | Lips (symmetry, color, dry/moist):<br>____________<br>Buccal mucosa (color/consistency/lesion/mass):<br>____________<br>Gums (color/lesions/swelling/bleeding/discharge):<br>____________<br>Odor from the mouth: ____________<br>Teeth (total number of teeth, color, tooth decay):<br>____________<br>Tongue (symmetry/color/texture/moisture): ____________<br>Hard and soft palate (color/lesion):<br>____________<br>Uvula (position/color):<br>____________<br>Tonsils (color/size/exudate):<br>____________<br>Pharynx (color/lesion/exudate):<br>____________ |

*Contd...*

<table>
<tr><th>Area/subjective data</th><th>Objective data</th></tr>
<tr><td>Thorax/Lungs</td><td>Is client on: Room air/oxygen/ventilator<br>If on oxygen support:<br>• Flow rate: ___<br>• Mode: ___<br>Endotracheal tube: Present/absent: ___<br>Thorax:<br>• Shape and symmetry: ___<br>• Position of sternum: ___<br>• Use of accessory muscles: ___<br>• Intercostal space (retraction/bulging): ___<br>• Respiratory rate: ___ Rhythm: ___<br>Dyspnea (shortness of breath):<br>• On rest: ___<br>• On exertion: ___<br>• Orthopnea: ___<br>• With expiratory/inspiratory wheezing: ___<br>Cough:<br>• Character (dry/hacking/brassy/wheezing): ___<br>• Time (morning/night): ___<br>Sputum:<br>• Color (colorless/yellowish/rust color/bright red/black):<br>___<br>• Odor: ___<br>Chest pain:<br>• Location (left/right side): ___<br>• Sharp/stabbing/intermittent/dull/aching/persistent: ___<br>• Duration: ___<br>Wheezing:<br>• Heard with/without stethoscope: ___<br>Hemoptysis: ___<br>Abnormal breath sounds (crackles/wheezing): ___<br>Trachea (position, mass):<br>___<br>___<br>___</td></tr>
</table>

*Contd...*

| Area/subjective data | Objective data |
|---|---|
| **Heart** | Chest pain: ______<br>______<br>• Referred pain (radiates to neck/arm/jaw/shoulders/hands/back/abdomen): ______<br>______<br>Palpitations: ______<br>Heart sounds: ______<br>Murmurs: ______ |
| **Breast and Axilla** | **Breast:**<br>• Size and symmetry: ______<br>• Color: ______<br>• Venous pattern: ______<br>• Thickening/edema: ______<br>• Ulceration/rashes: ______<br>• Scar: ______<br>**Areola:**<br>• Color: ______<br>• Lesion: ______<br>**Nipple:**<br>• Discharge: ______<br>• Retraction: ______<br>• Lesion: ______<br>**Axilla:**<br>• Tenderness: ______<br>• Axillary lymph nodes: ______ |

*Contd...*

| Area/subjective data | Objective data |
|---|---|
| **Abdomen** | Abdominal girth: ____________<br>Scars/lesions/rashes: ____________<br>Symmetry: ____________<br>Abdominal contour: ____________<br>Vomiting: ____________<br>____________<br>____________<br>**Changes in bowel habits and stool characteristics:** ____________<br>• Diarrhea: ____________<br>• Constipation: ____________<br>**Bowel sounds (normal/hypoactive/hyperactive/absent):** ____________<br>____________<br>**Tympany or dullness (during percussion):** ____________<br>____________<br>____________<br>Ascites: ____________<br>**Tenderness or swelling:**<br>• All quadrants: ____________<br>• Liver: ____________<br>• Spleen: ____________<br>• Appendix: ____________<br>• Kidney: ____________<br>• Urinary bladder: ____________ |

*Contd...*

| Area/subjective data | Objective data |
|---|---|
| **Genitalia** | Urinary catheter: Present/absent: ______<br>Urination (frequency, amount, color): ______<br>Urinary pattern (urgency, retention): ______<br>Burning micturition: ______<br>Hematuria: ______<br>**Male genitalia:**<br>• Penis: ______<br>• Scrotum: ______<br>• Inguinal area: ______<br>**Female genitalia:**<br>• Mons pubis: ______<br>• Labia majora: ______<br>• Urethra: ______<br>• Vagina: ______<br>• Cervix: ______ |
| **Anus and Rectum** | **Anus:**<br>• Anal opening area (redness, rashes, lump, ulcer, lesion, fissure, hemorrhoids): ______<br>______<br>Rectum (tenderness, smoothness, nodules): ______<br>______ |

*Contd...*

| Area/subjective data | Objective data |
|---|---|
| **Extremities** | Immobility: ______<br>Coordination: ______<br>Symmetry: ______<br>Capillary refill time: ______<br>Nails (cleanliness, color, clubbing, cyanosis): ______<br>______<br>______<br>Edema: ______<br>**Range of motion:**<br>• **Shoulder and arm:**<br>Flexion and hyperextension: ______<br>Adduction and abduction: ______<br>External and internal rotation: ______<br>• **Elbows:**<br>Flexion and extension: ______<br>Supination and pronation: ______<br>External and internal rotation: ______<br>• **Wrist:**<br>Flexion and extension: ______<br>• **Hands and fingers:**<br>Abduction and adduction: ______<br>Flexion and hyperextension: ______<br>• **Hips:**<br>Abduction and adduction: ______<br>Flexion and hyperextension: ______<br>• **Knees:**<br>Flexion and hyperextension: ______<br>• **Ankles and feet:**<br>Dorsiflexion and plantar flexion: ______<br>Eversion and inversion: ______<br>Abduction and adduction: ______<br>Varicose veins: ______ |

*Contd...*

| Area/subjective data | Objective data |
|---|---|
| **Skin** | **Color changes:**<br><br>• Pallor: ____________<br><br>• Jaundice: ____________<br><br>• Cyanosis: ____________<br><br>Temperature (warm/normal/cold and clammy): ____________<br>____________<br><br>Skin texture (rough/smooth): ____________<br><br>Skin turgor: ____________<br><br>Skin integrity (intact/bedsores): ____________<br>____________<br><br>Edema: ____________<br><br>Rash (location, itching): ____________<br><br>Lesions (macule/papule/vesicle/nodule/pustule/scar): ____________<br>____________ |

## EVALUATION CRITERIA FOR NURSING CARE PLAN

Name of the Student: ______________________________

Diagnosis of Patient: ______________________________

Ward/Unit: ____________________ Date of Submission: ____________________

| Sl. No. | Evaluation Criteria | Marks Obtained | Maximum Marks |
|---|---|---|---|
| 1 | Utilized therapeutic communication skills while interacting with patient and his/her family members | | 2 |
| 2 | Patient history | | 5 |
| 3 | Subjective and objective assessment | | 5 |
| 4 | Prioritized nursing diagnosis | | 2 |
| 5 | Goals | | 2 |
| 6 | Planning | | 2 |
| 7 | Implementation with rationale | | 2 |
| 8 | Evaluation | | 2 |
| 9 | Health education | | 2 |
| 10 | Timely submission | | 1 |
| **Total marks** | | | **25** |

**Remarks:** ______________________________

______________________________

______________________________

______________________________

**Signature of the Student** **Signature of the Clinical Supervisor**

**Date:** ____________ **Date:** ____________

## NURSING CARE PLAN–1

Date of collection of health history: ________ / ________ / ________

### I. BIOGRAPHICAL DATA OF THE PATIENT

Name of the patient: ______________________________

Fathers/Husband's name: ______________________________

Age: ______________ Gender: Male/Female ______________

Hospital: ______________________________

C.R./IP No.: ____________ Ward: ____________ Bed No.: ____________

Educational status: ______________ Occupation: ______________

Religion: ______________ Marital status: ______________

Address: ______________________________

______________________________

Date of admission: ______________________________

Treatment under Dr.: ______________________________

Diagnosis: ______________________________

Surgery performed, if any: ______________________________

Date of surgery performed: ______________________________

## II. CHIEF COMPLAINTS

At the time of admission: ______________________________

______________________________

______________________________

______________________________

At present:

______________________________

______________________________

______________________________

______________________________

______________________________

______________________________

## III. HISTORY OF PRESENT ILLNESS

(Includes details about chief complaints: Character, onset-sudden/gradual, location, duration, severity, pattern, aggravating factors, relieving factors, associated manifestations)

______________________________

______________________________

______________________________

______________________________

______________________________

______________________________

______________________________

______________________________

______________________________

______________________________

______________________________

## IV. PAST HEALTH HISTORY

(a) Childhood illness: ____________________

____________________

(b) Adult illnesses: ____________________

____________________

(c) Psychiatric illnesses: ____________________

____________________

(d) Previous hospitalizations: ____________________

____________________

____________________

(e) Previous surgical or diagnostic procedures: ____________________

____________________

(f) Allergies to foods/medications: ____________________

____________________

(g) Menstrual history (for female patient):

Last menstrual period (LMP) ____________ Menopausal: Yes/No ____________

Age at menarche: ____________ years. Menstruation: Regular/irregular duration: ____________

Does bleeding/spotting occur between periods: Yes/No ____________

Is pain associated with periods: ____________

(h) Past obstetrical history:

Have never been pregnant: ____________

Birth control/contraception: ____________

| **Number of pregnancies** | **Year** | **Pregnancy** (normal/miscarriage/abortion) | **Delivery** (normal/assisted/ cesarean section) | **Gender of baby** | **Puerperium** (normal/ complicated) |
|---|---|---|---|---|---|
| | | | | | |
| | | | | | |
| | | | | | |
| | | | | | |
| | | | | | |

## V. FAMILY HISTORY

(a) Family composition:

| Name | Age | Gender | Relationship with patient | Educational status | Occupation | Income | Health status |
|---|---|---|---|---|---|---|---|
| | | | | | | | |

(b) Family tree/genogram:

Key:

Male

Female

Patient

Deceased

(c) History of any recent death in family: Yes/No

Relationship with patient: ______________________ Age at death: ______________________

Cause of death: ______________________________________________

(d) History of any chronic illness in family:

(Hypertension, heart disease, diabetes, tuberculosis, asthma, renal disorder, arthritis, cancer, allergies, epilepsy, mental illness, etc.): Yes/No

If yes, give details: ______________________________________________

______________________________________________

______________________________________________

(e) History of any communicable disease in family: ______________________________

(f) History of any hereditary disease in family: ______________________________

## VI. LIFESTYLE

(a) Diet: Vegetarian/eggetarian/nonvegetarian/special diet: ______________________________

(b) Bowel and bladder habit: ______________________________

(c) Use of any addictive or illicit substance/drug (heroine/cocaine/alcohol/tobacco): Yes/No

(d) Sleeping pattern: ______________________________

(e) Exercise: ______________________________

(f) Recreation: ______________________________

(g) Religious belief: ______________________________

## VII. ENVIRONMENTAL HISTORY

(a) Physical-type of housing: ____________________

____________________

(b) Environmental hygiene: ____________________

____________________

(c) Source of drinking water: ____________________

____________________

(d) Presence of flies/mosquitoes/rodents: ____________________

____________________

(e) Disposal of excreta: ____________________

____________________

(f) Environmental pollution: ____________________

____________________

(g) Exposure to hazardous waste: ____________________

____________________

# GENERAL PHYSICAL EXAMINATION

## I. GENERAL APPEARANCE

Level of consciousness (conscious/semiconscious/unconscious/coma): ______________________

Orientation (time, place and person): ______________________

______________________

______________________

Activity (active/dull): ______________________

Body built (average/thin/obese): ______________________

Look (anxious/depressed): ______________________

Posture (Body curves: Lordosis/kyphosis/scoliosis): ______________________

## II. ANTHROPOMETRIC MEASUREMENT

Height: ______________ Weight: ______________ BMI: ______________

[Body mass index; BMI = Weight (in kilograms)/Height$^2$ (in meters)]

## III. VITAL SIGNS

| Date/vitals | Temperature (in C°/F°) | Pulse (beats/min) | Respiration (breaths/min) | Blood pressure (in mm Hg) |
|---|---|---|---|---|
| | | | | |
| | | | | |
| | | | | |
| | | | | |
| | | | | |
| | | | | |
| | | | | |

| Area/subjective data | Objective data |
|---|---|
| **Head and Neck** | **Scalp:**<br>• Cleanliness: ____________<br>• Abrasions/wound: ____________<br>____________<br>**Hairs:**<br>• Color: ____________<br>• Texture (fine/coarse/brittle/dull): ____________<br>• Distribution (hair loss): ____________<br>• Dandruff: ____________<br>• Pediculi or any other infection: ____________<br>**Face (pale, puffiness, expressions, enlargement of parotid glands):** ____________<br>____________<br>**Neck:**<br>• Lump or mass: ____________<br>• Lymphadenopathy: ____________<br>• Range of motion (flexion, extension, rotation):<br>____________<br>____________<br>• Jugular venous pulses: ____________<br>**Thyroid gland (landmarks, lump):**<br>____________<br>____________ |

*Contd...*

| Area/subjective data | Objective data |
|---|---|
| **Eyes** | **Eyelids:**<br>• Position (ptosis/lid retraction): ____________<br>**Lid margin:**<br>• Edema: ____________<br>• Erythema: ____________<br>• Lesions: ____________<br>**Sclera:**<br>____________<br>____________<br>**Conjunctiva:**<br>____________<br>____________<br>**Pupils:**<br>• Color: ____________<br>• Pupillary response: ____________<br>____________<br>____________<br>**Extraocular movements:**<br>____________<br>____________<br>Use of spectacles/contact lens: ____________<br>____________<br>Visual acuity: ____________<br>____________ |

*Contd...*

| Area/subjective data | Objective data |
|---|---|
| **Ears** | **Use of hearing aids:** ______<br><br>**Auricle (deformity, lesion, discharge, size, symmetry, angle of attachment to head):** ______<br>______<br>______<br>______<br><br>**Mastoid area (tenderness):** ______<br>______<br><br>**External auditory canal (discharge/cerumen/fluid/blood, nodule):** ______<br>______<br><br>**Tympanic membrane (color):** ______<br><br>**Hearing acuity:** ______<br><br>• Whisper test: ______<br><br>• Weber test: ______<br><br>• Rinne test: ______ |

*Contd...*

| Area/subjective data | Objective data |
|---|---|
| **Nose and Sinuses** | **External nose:**<br>• Lesions: ______<br>• Asymmetry: ______<br>• Inflammation: ______<br>**Internal structures of nose:**<br>• Nasal mucosa (color/swelling/exudates/bleeding/polyps):<br>______<br>______<br>______<br>______<br>Nasal septum (central/deviated): ______<br>**Sinuses:**<br>• Frontal sinuses: ______<br>• Maxillary sinuses: ______ |
| **Mouth and Pharynx** | Lips (symmetry, color, dry/moist):<br>______<br>Buccal mucosa (color/consistency/lesion/mass):<br>______<br>Gums (color/lesions/swelling/bleeding/discharge):<br>______<br>Odor from the mouth: ______<br>Teeth (total number of teeth, color, tooth decay):<br>______<br>Tongue (symmetry/color/texture/moisture): ______<br>Hard and soft palate (color/lesion):<br>______<br>Uvula (position/color):<br>______<br>Tonsils (color/size/exudate):<br>______<br>Pharynx (color/lesion/exudate):<br>______ |

*Contd...*

| Area/subjective data | Objective data |
|---|---|
| **Thorax/Lungs** | **Is client on: Room air/oxygen/ventilator**<br>If on oxygen support:<br>• Flow rate: ____________<br>• Mode: ____________<br>Endotracheal tube: Present/absent: ____________<br>**Thorax:**<br>• Shape and symmetry: ____________<br>• Position of sternum: ____________<br>• Use of accessory muscles: ____________<br>• Intercostal space (retraction/bulging): ____________<br>• Respiratory rate: ____________ Rhythm: ____________<br>**Dyspnea (shortness of breath):**<br>• On rest: ____________<br>• On exertion: ____________<br>• Orthopnea: ____________<br>• With expiratory/inspiratory wheezing: ____________<br>**Cough:**<br>• Character (dry/hacking/brassy/wheezing): ____________<br>• Time (morning/night): ____________<br>**Sputum:**<br>• Color (colorless/yellowish/rust color/bright red/black):<br>____________<br>• Odor: ____________<br>**Chest pain:**<br>• Location (left/right side): ____________<br>• Sharp/stabbing/intermittent/dull/aching/persistent: ____________<br>• Duration: ____________<br>**Wheezing:**<br>• Heard with/without stethoscope: ____________<br>Hemoptysis: ____________<br>Abnormal breath sounds (crackles/wheezing): ____________<br>**Trachea (position, mass):**<br>____________<br>____________<br>____________ |

*Contd...*

| Area/subjective data | Objective data |
|---|---|
| **Heart** | Chest pain: ______<br>______<br>• Referred pain (radiates to neck/arm/jaw/shoulders/hands/back/abdomen): ______<br>______<br>Palpitations: ______<br>Heart sounds: ______<br>Murmurs: ______ |
| **Breast and Axilla** | **Breast:**<br>• Size and symmetry: ______<br>• Color: ______<br>• Venous pattern: ______<br>• Thickening/edema: ______<br>• Ulceration/rashes: ______<br>• Scar: ______<br>**Areola:**<br>• Color: ______<br>• Lesion: ______<br>**Nipple:**<br>• Discharge: ______<br>• Retraction: ______<br>• Lesion: ______<br>**Axilla:**<br>• Tenderness: ______<br>• Axillary lymph nodes: ______ |

*Contd...*

| Area/subjective data | Objective data |
|---|---|
| **Abdomen** | Abdominal girth: ______<br>Scars/lesions/rashes: ______<br>Symmetry: ______<br>Abdominal contour: ______<br>Vomiting: ______<br>______<br>______<br>**Changes in bowel habits and stool characteristics:** ______<br>• Diarrhea: ______<br>• Constipation: ______<br>**Bowel sounds (normal/hypoactive/hyperactive/absent):** ______<br>______<br>**Tympany or dullness (during percussion):** ______<br>______<br>______<br>Ascites: ______<br>**Tenderness or swelling:**<br>• All quadrants: ______<br>• Liver: ______<br>• Spleen: ______<br>• Appendix: ______<br>• Kidney: ______<br>• Urinary bladder: ______ |

*Contd...*

| Area/subjective data | Objective data |
|---|---|
| **Genitalia** | Urinary catheter: Present/absent: ____<br>Urination (frequency, amount, color): ____<br>Urinary pattern (urgency, retention): ____<br>Burning micturition: ____<br>Hematuria: ____<br>**Male genitalia:**<br>• Penis: ____<br>• Scrotum: ____<br>• Inguinal area: ____<br>**Female genitalia:**<br>• Mons pubis: ____<br>• Labia majora: ____<br>• Urethra: ____<br>• Vagina: ____<br>• Cervix: ____ |
| **Anus and Rectum** | **Anus:**<br>• Anal opening area (redness, rashes, lump, ulcer, lesion, fissure, hemorrhoids): ____<br>____<br>Rectum (tenderness, smoothness, nodules): ____<br>____ |

*Contd...*

| Area/subjective data | Objective data |
|---|---|
| **Extremities** | Immobility: ______<br>Coordination: ______<br>Symmetry: ______<br>Capillary refill time: ______<br>Nails (cleanliness, color, clubbing, cyanosis): ______<br>______<br>______<br>Edema: ______<br>**Range of motion:**<br>• **Shoulder and arm:**<br>Flexion and hyperextension: ______<br>Adduction and abduction: ______<br>External and internal rotation: ______<br>• **Elbows:**<br>Flexion and extension: ______<br>Supination and pronation: ______<br>External and internal rotation: ______<br>• **Wrist:**<br>Flexion and extension: ______<br>• **Hands and fingers:**<br>Abduction and adduction: ______<br>Flexion and hyperextension: ______<br>• **Hips:**<br>Abduction and adduction: ______<br>Flexion and hyperextension: ______<br>• **Knees:**<br>Flexion and hyperextension: ______<br>• **Ankles and feet:**<br>Dorsiflexion and plantar flexion: ______<br>Eversion and inversion: ______<br>Abduction and adduction: ______<br>Varicose veins: ______ |

*Contd...*

| Area/subjective data | Objective data |
|---|---|
| **Skin** | **Color changes:**<br>• Pallor: ____________<br>• Jaundice: ____________<br>• Cyanosis: ____________<br>Temperature (warm/normal/cold and clammy): ____________<br>____________<br>Skin texture (rough/smooth): ____________<br>Skin turgor: ____________<br>Skin integrity (intact/bedsores): ____________<br>____________<br>Edema: ____________<br>Rash (location, itching): ____________<br>Lesions (macule/papule/vesicle/nodule/pustule/scar): ____________<br>____________ |

## LABORATORY INVESTIGATIONS

| Date | Investigations | Patients Value | Normal Value | Remarks |
|---|---|---|---|---|
| | | | | |

**Radiological investigations:**

Date:________________

Findings: ________________________________________________________

## MEDICATION

| Trade Name | Pharmaceutical Name | Dose | Route | Frequency | Action |
|---|---|---|---|---|---|
| | | | | | |

# INTAKE AND OUTPUT CHART

Date:____________/____________/____________

| Time | Intake (in mL) | | | | Total | Time | Output (in mL) | | | | | Total |
|---|---|---|---|---|---|---|---|---|---|---|---|---|
| | Oral | IV | NG | Blood | | | Urine | Stool | NG aspiration | Vomiting | Drainage | |
| | | | | | | | | | | | | |
| | | | | | | | | | | | | |
| | | | | | | | | | | | | |
| | | | | | | | | | | | | |
| | | | | | | | | | | | | |
| | | | | | | | | | | | | |
| | | | | | | | | | | | | |
| | | | | | | | | | | | | |
| | | | | | | | | | | | | |
| | | | | | | | | | | | | |
| | | | | | | | | | | | | |
| | | | | | | | | | | | | |
| | | | | | | | | | | | | |
| | | | | | | | | | | | | |
| | | | | | | | | | | | | |
| | | | | | | | | | | | | |
| | | | | | | | | | | | | |
| | | | | | | | | | | | | |
| | | | | | | | | | | | | |
| | | | | | | | | | | | | |
| | | | | | | | | | | | | |
| | | | | | | | | | | | | |
| | | | | | | | | | | | | |
| | | | | | | | | | | | | |
| Total intake (in mL) | | | | | | Total output (in mL) | | | | | | |

Balance: +/– ______________________

## NURSING MANAGEMENT

**Identified nursing needs and problems of patient:**

**Nursing diagnosis:**

**Short-term goals:**

**Long-term goals:**

## NURSING CARE PLAN

| Assessment (subjective and objective) | Nursing diagnosis | Goal | Planning | Implementation | Rationale | Evaluation |
|---|---|---|---|---|---|---|
| | | | | | | |

| Assessment (subjective and objective) | Nursing diagnosis | Goal | Planning | Implementation | Rationale | Evaluation |
|---|---|---|---|---|---|---|
| | | | | | | |

| Assessment (subjective and objective) | Nursing diagnosis | Goal | Planning | Implementation | Rationale | Evaluation |
|---|---|---|---|---|---|---|
| | | | | | | |

| Assessment (subjective and objective) | Nursing diagnosis | Goal | Planning | Implementation | Rationale | Evaluation |
|---|---|---|---|---|---|---|
| | | | | | | |

| Assessment (subjective and objective) | Nursing diagnosis | Goal | Planning | Implementation | Rationale | Evaluation |
|---|---|---|---|---|---|---|
| | | | | | | |

| Assessment (subjective and objective) | Nursing diagnosis | Goal | Planning | Implementation | Rationale | Evaluation |
|---|---|---|---|---|---|---|
| | | | | | | |

## HEALTH EDUCATION

1. **Disease Condition**

2. **Personal Hygiene**

3. **Diet**

4. **Lifestyle Modification**

5. **Medication**

6. **Follow-up Care**

## EVALUATION CRITERIA FOR NURSING CARE PLAN

Name of the Student: ____________________

Diagnosis of Patient: ____________________

Ward/Unit: ____________________ Date of Submission: ____________________

| Sl. No. | Evaluation Criteria | Marks Obtained | Maximum Marks |
|---|---|---|---|
| 1 | Utilized therapeutic communication skills while interacting with patient and his/her family members | | 2 |
| 2 | Patient history | | 5 |
| 3 | Subjective and objective assessment | | 5 |
| 4 | Prioritized nursing diagnosis | | 2 |
| 5 | Goals | | 2 |
| 6 | Planning | | 2 |
| 7 | Implementation with rationale | | 2 |
| 8 | Evaluation | | 2 |
| 9 | Health education | | 2 |
| 10 | Timely submission | | 1 |
| **Total marks** | | | **25** |

**Remarks:** ____________________

____________________

____________________

**Signature of the Student**

**Signature of the Clinical Supervisor**

**Date:** ____________________

**Date:** ____________________

# NURSING CARE PLAN–2

Date of collection of health history: _________ / _________ / _________

## I. BIOGRAPHICAL DATA OF THE PATIENT

Name of the patient: ____________________

Fathers/Husband's name: ____________________

Age: ____________________ Gender: Male/Female ____________________

Hospital: ____________________

C.R./IP No.: ____________ Ward: ____________ Bed No.: ____________

Educational status: ____________________ Occupation: ____________________

Religion: ____________________ Marital status: ____________________

Address: ____________________

____________________

Date of admission: ____________________

Treatment under Dr.: ____________________

Diagnosis: ____________________

Surgery performed, if any: ____________________

Date of surgery performed: ____________________

## II. CHIEF COMPLAINTS

At the time of admission: ______________________________

______________________________

______________________________

______________________________

At present:

______________________________

______________________________

______________________________

______________________________

______________________________

______________________________

## III. HISTORY OF PRESENT ILLNESS

(Includes details about chief complaints: Character, onset-sudden/gradual, location, duration, severity, pattern, aggravating factors, relieving factors, associated manifestations)

______________________________

______________________________

______________________________

______________________________

______________________________

______________________________

______________________________

______________________________

______________________________

______________________________

______________________________

## IV. PAST HEALTH HISTORY

(a) Childhood illness: ______________________________

______________________________

(b) Adult illnesses: ______________________________

______________________________

(c) Psychiatric illnesses: ______________________________

______________________________

(d) Previous hospitalizations: ______________________________

______________________________

______________________________

(e) Previous surgical or diagnostic procedures: ______________________________

______________________________

(f) Allergies to foods/medications: ______________________________

______________________________

(g) Menstrual history (for female patient):

Last menstrual period (LMP) ______________ Menopausal: Yes/No ______________

Age at menarche: ______________ years. Menstruation: Regular/irregular duration: ______________

Does bleeding/spotting occur between periods: Yes/No ______________

Is pain associated with periods: ______________

(h) Past obstetrical history:

Have never been pregnant: ______________

Birth control/contraception: ______________

| Number of pregnancies | Year | Pregnancy (normal/miscarriage/abortion) | Delivery (normal/assisted/ cesarean section) | Gender of baby | Puerperium (normal/ complicated) |
|---|---|---|---|---|---|
| | | | | | |
| | | | | | |
| | | | | | |
| | | | | | |
| | | | | | |

## V. FAMILY HISTORY

(a) Family composition:

| Name | Age | Gender | Relationship with patient | Educational status | Occupation | Income | Health status |
|---|---|---|---|---|---|---|---|
| | | | | | | | |

(b) Family tree/genogram:

Key:

| | |
|---|---|
| Male | ○ |
| Female | □ |
| Patient | → |
| Deceased | ■ ● |

(c) History of any recent death in family: Yes/No

Relationship with patient: ______________________ Age at death: ______________________

Cause of death: ________________________________________________

(d) History of any chronic illness in family:

(Hypertension, heart disease, diabetes, tuberculosis, asthma, renal disorder, arthritis, cancer, allergies, epilepsy, mental illness, etc.): Yes/No

If yes, give details: ________________________________________________

________________________________________________

________________________________________________

(e) History of any communicable disease in family: ______________________________

______________________________

______________________________

(f) History of any hereditary disease in family: ______________________________

______________________________

______________________________

## VI. LIFESTYLE

(a) Diet: Vegetarian/eggetarian/nonvegetarian/special diet: ______________________________

______________________________

(b) Bowel and bladder habit: ______________________________

______________________________

(c) Use of any addictive or illicit substance/drug (heroine/cocaine/alcohol/tobacco): Yes/No

______________________________

______________________________

______________________________

______________________________

(d) Sleeping pattern: ______________________________

______________________________

(e) Exercise: ______________________________

______________________________

(f) Recreation: ______________________________

______________________________

(g) Religious belief: ______________________________

______________________________

## VII. ENVIRONMENTAL HISTORY

(a) Physical-type of housing: ______________________________

______________________________

(b) Environmental hygiene: ______________________________

______________________________

(c) Source of drinking water: ______________________________

______________________________

(d) Presence of flies/mosquitoes/rodents: ______________________________

______________________________

(e) Disposal of excreta: ______________________________

______________________________

(f) Environmental pollution: ______________________________

______________________________

(g) Exposure to hazardous waste: ______________________________

______________________________

# GENERAL PHYSICAL EXAMINATION

## I. GENERAL APPEARANCE

Level of consciousness (conscious/semiconscious/unconscious/coma): ____________________

Orientation (time, place and person): ____________________

____________________

____________________

Activity (active/dull): ____________________

Body built (average/thin/obese): ____________________

Look (anxious/depressed): ____________________

Posture (Body curves: Lordosis/kyphosis/scoliosis): ____________________

## II. ANTHROPOMETRIC MEASUREMENT

Height: ______________ Weight: ______________ BMI: ______________

[Body mass index; BMI = Weight (in kilograms)/Height$^2$ (in meters)]

## III. VITAL SIGNS

| Date/vitals | Temperature (in C°/F°) | Pulse (beats/min) | Respiration (breaths/min) | Blood pressure (in mm Hg) |
|---|---|---|---|---|
| | | | | |
| | | | | |
| | | | | |
| | | | | |
| | | | | |
| | | | | |
| | | | | |

| Area/subjective data | Objective data |
|---|---|
| **Head and Neck** | **Scalp:**<br>• Cleanliness: ____________<br>• Abrasions/wound: ____________<br>____________<br>**Hairs:**<br>• Color: ____________<br>• Texture (fine/coarse/brittle/dull): ____________<br>• Distribution (hair loss): ____________<br>• Dandruff: ____________<br>• Pediculi or any other infection: ____________<br>**Face (pale, puffiness, expressions, enlargement of parotid glands):** ____________<br>____________<br>**Neck:**<br>• Lump or mass: ____________<br>• Lymphadenopathy: ____________<br>• Range of motion (flexion, extension, rotation):<br>____________<br>____________<br>• Jugular venous pulses: ____________<br>**Thyroid gland (landmarks, lump):**<br>____________<br>____________ |

*Contd...*

<table>
<tr><th>Area/subjective data</th><th>Objective data</th></tr>
<tr><td>Eyes</td><td>Eyelids:<br>• Position (ptosis/lid retraction): ____________________<br>Lid margin:<br>• Edema: ____________________<br>• Erythema: ____________________<br>• Lesions: ____________________<br>Sclera:<br>____________________<br>____________________<br>Conjunctiva:<br>____________________<br>____________________<br>Pupils:<br>• Color: ____________________<br>• Pupillary response: ____________________<br>____________________<br>____________________<br>Extraocular movements:<br>____________________<br>____________________<br>Use of spectacles/contact lens: ____________________<br>____________________<br>Visual acuity: ____________________<br>____________________</td></tr>
</table>

*Contd...*

| Area/subjective data | Objective data |
|---|---|
| **Ears** | **Use of hearing aids:** ______<br><br>**Auricle (deformity, lesion, discharge, size, symmetry, angle of attachment to head):** ______<br>______<br>______<br>______<br><br>**Mastoid area (tenderness):** ______<br>______<br><br>**External auditory canal (discharge/cerumen/fluid/blood, nodule):** ______<br>______<br><br>**Tympanic membrane (color):** ______<br><br>**Hearing acuity:** ______<br><br>• Whisper test: ______<br><br>• Weber test: ______<br><br>• Rinne test: ______ |

*Contd...*

| Area/subjective data | Objective data |
|---|---|
| **Nose and Sinuses** | **External nose:**<br>• Lesions: ______<br>• Asymmetry: ______<br>• Inflammation: ______<br>**Internal structures of nose:**<br>• Nasal mucosa (color/swelling/exudates/bleeding/polyps):<br>______<br>______<br>______<br>______<br>Nasal septum (central/deviated): ______<br>**Sinuses:**<br>• Frontal sinuses: ______<br>• Maxillary sinuses: ______ |
| **Mouth and Pharynx** | Lips (symmetry, color, dry/moist):<br>______<br>Buccal mucosa (color/consistency/lesion/mass):<br>______<br>Gums (color/lesions/swelling/bleeding/discharge):<br>______<br>Odor from the mouth: ______<br>Teeth (total number of teeth, color, tooth decay):<br>______<br>Tongue (symmetry/color/texture/moisture): ______<br>Hard and soft palate (color/lesion):<br>______<br>Uvula (position/color):<br>______<br>Tonsils (color/size/exudate):<br>______<br>Pharynx (color/lesion/exudate):<br>______ |

*Contd...*

| Area/subjective data | Objective data |
|---|---|
| **Thorax/Lungs** | **Is client on: Room air/oxygen/ventilator**<br>If on oxygen support:<br>• Flow rate: ____________<br>• Mode: ____________<br>Endotracheal tube: Present/absent: ____________<br>**Thorax:**<br>• Shape and symmetry: ____________<br>• Position of sternum: ____________<br>• Use of accessory muscles: ____________<br>• Intercostal space (retraction/bulging): ____________<br>• Respiratory rate: ____________ Rhythm: ____________<br>**Dyspnea (shortness of breath):**<br>• On rest: ____________<br>• On exertion: ____________<br>• Orthopnea: ____________<br>• With expiratory/inspiratory wheezing: ____________<br>**Cough:**<br>• Character (dry/hacking/brassy/wheezing): ____________<br>• Time (morning/night): ____________<br>**Sputum:**<br>• Color (colorless/yellowish/rust color/bright red/black):<br>____________<br>• Odor: ____________<br>**Chest pain:**<br>• Location (left/right side): ____________<br>• Sharp/stabbing/intermittent/dull/aching/persistent: ____________<br>• Duration: ____________<br>**Wheezing:**<br>• Heard with/without stethoscope: ____________<br>Hemoptysis: ____________<br>Abnormal breath sounds (crackles/wheezing): ____________<br>**Trachea (position, mass):**<br>____________<br>____________<br>____________ |

*Contd...*

| Area/subjective data | Objective data |
|---|---|
| **Heart** | Chest pain: ________________<br>________________<br>• Referred pain (radiates to neck/arm/jaw/shoulders/hands/back/abdomen): ________________<br>________________<br>Palpitations: ________________<br>Heart sounds: ________________<br>Murmurs: ________________ |
| **Breast and Axilla** | **Breast:**<br>• Size and symmetry: ________________<br>• Color: ________________<br>• Venous pattern: ________________<br>• Thickening/edema: ________________<br>• Ulceration/rashes: ________________<br>• Scar: ________________<br>**Areola:**<br>• Color: ________________<br>• Lesion: ________________<br>**Nipple:**<br>• Discharge: ________________<br>• Retraction: ________________<br>• Lesion: ________________<br>**Axilla:**<br>• Tenderness: ________________<br>• Axillary lymph nodes: ________________ |

*Contd...*

<table>
<tr><th>Area/subjective data</th><th>Objective data</th></tr>
<tr><td>Abdomen</td><td>Abdominal girth: ______<br>Scars/lesions/rashes: ______<br>Symmetry: ______<br>Abdominal contour: ______<br>Vomiting: ______<br>______<br>______<br>Changes in bowel habits and stool characteristics: ______<br>• Diarrhea: ______<br>• Constipation: ______<br>Bowel sounds (normal/hypoactive/hyperactive/absent): ______<br>______<br>Tympany or dullness (during percussion): ______<br>______<br>______<br>Ascites: ______<br>Tenderness or swelling:<br>• All quadrants: ______<br>• Liver:<br>• Spleen: ______<br>• Appendix: ______<br>• Kidney: ______<br>• Urinary bladder: ______</td></tr>
</table>

*Contd...*

| Area/subjective data | Objective data |
|---|---|
| **Genitalia** | Urinary catheter: Present/absent: ______<br>Urination (frequency, amount, color): ______<br>Urinary pattern (urgency, retention): ______<br>Burning micturition: ______<br>Hematuria: ______<br>**Male genitalia:**<br>• Penis: ______<br>• Scrotum: ______<br>• Inguinal area: ______<br>**Female genitalia:**<br>• Mons pubis: ______<br>• Labia majora: ______<br>• Urethra: ______<br>• Vagina: ______<br>• Cervix: ______ |
| **Anus and Rectum** | **Anus:**<br>• Anal opening area (redness, rashes, lump, ulcer, lesion, fissure, hemorrhoids): ______<br>______<br>Rectum (tenderness, smoothness, nodules): ______<br>______ |

*Contd...*

| Area/subjective data | Objective data |
|---|---|
| **Extremities** | Immobility: ______<br>Coordination: ______<br>Symmetry: ______<br>Capillary refill time: ______<br>Nails (cleanliness, color, clubbing, cyanosis): ______<br>______<br>______<br>Edema: ______<br>**Range of motion:**<br>• **Shoulder and arm:**<br>Flexion and hyperextension: ______<br>Adduction and abduction: ______<br>External and internal rotation: ______<br>• **Elbows:**<br>Flexion and extension: ______<br>Supination and pronation: ______<br>External and internal rotation: ______<br>• **Wrist:**<br>Flexion and extension: ______<br>• **Hands and fingers:**<br>Abduction and adduction: ______<br>Flexion and hyperextension: ______<br>• **Hips:**<br>Abduction and adduction: ______<br>Flexion and hyperextension: ______<br>• **Knees:**<br>Flexion and hyperextension: ______<br>• **Ankles and feet:**<br>Dorsiflexion and plantar flexion: ______<br>Eversion and inversion: ______<br>Abduction and adduction: ______<br>Varicose veins: ______ |

*Contd...*

| Area/subjective data | Objective data |
|---|---|
| **Skin** | **Color changes:**<br>• Pallor: ____________<br>• Jaundice: ____________<br>• Cyanosis: ____________<br>Temperature (warm/normal/cold and clammy): ____________<br>____________<br>Skin texture (rough/smooth): ____________<br>Skin turgor: ____________<br>Skin integrity (intact/bedsores): ____________<br>____________<br>Edema: ____________<br>Rash (location, itching): ____________<br>Lesions (macule/papule/vesicle/nodule/pustule/scar): ____________<br>____________ |

## LABORATORY INVESTIGATIONS

| Date | Investigations | Patient's Value | Normal Value | Remarks |
|---|---|---|---|---|
| | | | | |

**Radiological investigations:**

Date:________________

Findings: ____________________________________________________________

## MEDICATION

| Trade Name | Pharmaceutical Name | Dose | Route | Frequency | Action |
|---|---|---|---|---|---|
| | | | | | |

## INTAKE AND OUTPUT CHART

Date:__________ /__________ / __________

| Time | Intake (in mL) | | | | Total | Time | Output (in mL) | | | | | Total |
|---|---|---|---|---|---|---|---|---|---|---|---|---|
| | Oral | IV | NG | Blood | | | Urine | Stool | NG aspiration | Vomiting | Drainage | |
| | | | | | | | | | | | | |
| | | | | | | | | | | | | |
| | | | | | | | | | | | | |
| | | | | | | | | | | | | |
| | | | | | | | | | | | | |
| | | | | | | | | | | | | |
| | | | | | | | | | | | | |
| | | | | | | | | | | | | |
| | | | | | | | | | | | | |
| | | | | | | | | | | | | |
| | | | | | | | | | | | | |
| | | | | | | | | | | | | |
| | | | | | | | | | | | | |
| | | | | | | | | | | | | |
| | | | | | | | | | | | | |
| | | | | | | | | | | | | |
| | | | | | | | | | | | | |
| | | | | | | | | | | | | |
| | | | | | | | | | | | | |
| | | | | | | | | | | | | |
| | | | | | | | | | | | | |
| | | | | | | | | | | | | |
| | | | | | | | | | | | | |
| | | | | | | | | | | | | |
| Total intake (in mL) | | | | | | Total output (in mL) | | | | | | |

Balance: +/– ____________________

## NURSING MANAGEMENT

**Identified nursing needs and problems of patient:**

**Nursing diagnosis:**

**Short-term goals:**

**Long-term goals:**

## NURSING CARE PLAN

| Assessment (subjective and objective) | Nursing diagnosis | Goal | Planning | Implementation | Rationale | Evaluation |
|---|---|---|---|---|---|---|
| | | | | | | |

| Assessment (subjective and objective) | Nursing diagnosis | Goal | Planning | Implementation | Rationale | Evaluation |
|---|---|---|---|---|---|---|
| | | | | | | |

| Assessment (subjective and objective) | Nursing diagnosis | Goal | Planning | Implementation | Rationale | Evaluation |
|---|---|---|---|---|---|---|
| | | | | | | |

| Assessment (subjective and objective) | Nursing diagnosis | Goal | Planning | Implementation | Rationale | Evaluation |
|---|---|---|---|---|---|---|
| | | | | | | |

| Assessment (subjective and objective) | Nursing diagnosis | Goal | Planning | Implementation | Rationale | Evaluation |
|---|---|---|---|---|---|---|
| | | | | | | |

| Assessment (subjective and objective) | Nursing diagnosis | Goal | Planning | Implementation | Rationale | Evaluation |
|---|---|---|---|---|---|---|
| | | | | | | |

## HEALTH EDUCATION

**1. Disease Condition**

**2. Personal Hygiene**

**3. Diet**

**4. Lifestyle Modification**

**5. Medication**

**6. Follow-up Care**

# EVALUATION CRITERIA FOR NURSING CARE PLAN

Name of the Student: ______________________________

Diagnosis of Patient: ______________________________

Ward/Unit: ____________________ Date of Submission: ____________________

| Sl. No. | Evaluation Criteria | Marks Obtained | Maximum Marks |
|---|---|---|---|
| 1 | Utilized therapeutic communication skills while interacting with patient and his/her family members | | 2 |
| 2 | Patient history | | 5 |
| 3 | Subjective and objective assessment | | 5 |
| 4 | Prioritized nursing diagnosis | | 2 |
| 5 | Goals | | 2 |
| 6 | Planning | | 2 |
| 7 | Implementation with rationale | | 2 |
| 8 | Evaluation | | 2 |
| 9 | Health education | | 2 |
| 10 | Timely submission | | 1 |
| **Total marks** | | | **25** |

**Remarks:** ______________________________

______________________________

______________________________

______________________ ______________________

**Signature of the Student** **Signature of the Clinical Supervisor**

**Date:** ____________ **Date:** ____________

# NURSING CARE PLAN–3

Date of collection of health history: ________ / ________ / ________

## I. BIOGRAPHICAL DATA OF THE PATIENT

Name of the patient: ____________________

Fathers/Husband's name: ____________________

Age: ____________________ Gender: Male/Female ____________________

Hospital: ____________________

C.R./IP No.: ____________ Ward: ____________ Bed No.: ____________

Educational status: ____________________ Occupation: ____________________

Religion: ____________________ Marital status: ____________________

Address: ____________________

____________________

Date of admission: ____________________

Treatment under Dr.: ____________________

Diagnosis: ____________________

Surgery performed, if any: ____________________

Date of surgery performed: ____________________

## II. CHIEF COMPLAINTS

At the time of admission: ____________________________________________

____________________________________________

____________________________________________

____________________________________________

At present:

____________________________________________

____________________________________________

____________________________________________

____________________________________________

____________________________________________

____________________________________________

## III. HISTORY OF PRESENT ILLNESS

(Includes details about chief complaints: Character, onset-sudden/gradual, location, duration, severity, pattern, aggravating factors, relieving factors, associated manifestations)

____________________________________________

____________________________________________

____________________________________________

____________________________________________

____________________________________________

____________________________________________

____________________________________________

____________________________________________

____________________________________________

____________________________________________

____________________________________________

## IV. PAST HEALTH HISTORY

(a) Childhood illness: ______________________________

______________________________

(b) Adult illnesses: ______________________________

______________________________

(c) Psychiatric illnesses: ______________________________

______________________________

(d) Previous hospitalizations: ______________________________

______________________________

______________________________

(e) Previous surgical or diagnostic procedures: ______________________________

______________________________

(f) Allergies to foods/medications: ______________________________

______________________________

(g) Menstrual history (for female patient):

Last menstrual period (LMP) ______________ Menopausal: Yes/No ______________

Age at menarche: ______________ years. Menstruation: Regular/irregular duration: ______________

Does bleeding/spotting occur between periods: Yes/No ______________

Is pain associated with periods: ______________________________

(h) Past obstetrical history:

Have never been pregnant: ______________________________

Birth control/contraception: ______________________________

| **Number of pregnancies** | **Year** | **Pregnancy** (normal/miscarriage/abortion) | **Delivery** (normal/assisted/ cesarean section) | **Gender of baby** | **Puerperium** (normal/ complicated) |
|---|---|---|---|---|---|
| | | | | | |
| | | | | | |
| | | | | | |
| | | | | | |
| | | | | | |

## V. FAMILY HISTORY

(a) Family composition:

| Name | Age | Gender | Relationship with patient | Educational status | Occupation | Income | Health status |
|---|---|---|---|---|---|---|---|
| | | | | | | | |

(b) Family tree/genogram:

Key:

Male ○

Female □

Patient →

Deceased ■ ●

(c) History of any recent death in family: Yes/No

Relationship with patient: ______________________ Age at death: ______________________

Cause of death: ____________________________________________

(d) History of any chronic illness in family:

(Hypertension, heart disease, diabetes, tuberculosis, asthma, renal disorder, arthritis, cancer, allergies, epilepsy, mental illness, etc.): Yes/No

If yes, give details: ____________________________________________

____________________________________________

____________________________________________

(e) History of any communicable disease in family: ______________________

______________________

______________________

(f) History of any hereditary disease in family: ______________________

______________________

______________________

## VI. LIFESTYLE

(a) Diet: Vegetarian/eggetarian/nonvegetarian/special diet: ______________________

______________________

(b) Bowel and bladder habit: ______________________

______________________

(c) Use of any addictive or illicit substance/drug (heroine/cocaine/alcohol/tobacco): Yes/No

______________________

______________________

______________________

______________________

(d) Sleeping pattern: ______________________

______________________

(e) Exercise: ______________________

______________________

(f) Recreation: ______________________

______________________

(g) Religious belief: ______________________

______________________

## VII. ENVIRONMENTAL HISTORY

(a) Physical-type of housing: ______________________________

______________________________

(b) Environmental hygiene: ______________________________

______________________________

(c) Source of drinking water: ______________________________

______________________________

(d) Presence of flies/mosquitoes/rodents: ______________________________

______________________________

(e) Disposal of excreta: ______________________________

______________________________

(f) Environmental pollution: ______________________________

______________________________

(g) Exposure to hazardous waste: ______________________________

______________________________

# GENERAL PHYSICAL EXAMINATION

## I. GENERAL APPEARANCE

Level of consciousness (conscious/semiconscious/unconscious/coma): ____________________

Orientation (time, place and person): ____________________

____________________

____________________

Activity (active/dull): ____________________

Body built (average/thin/obese): ____________________

Look (anxious/depressed): ____________________

Posture (Body curves: Lordosis/kyphosis/scoliosis): ____________________

## II. ANTHROPOMETRIC MEASUREMENT

Height: ______________ Weight: ______________ BMI: ______________

[Body mass index; BMI = Weight (in kilograms)/Height$^2$ (in meters)]

## III. VITAL SIGNS

| Date/vitals | Temperature (in C°/F°) | Pulse (beats/min) | Respiration (breaths/min) | Blood pressure (in mm Hg) |
|---|---|---|---|---|
| | | | | |
| | | | | |
| | | | | |
| | | | | |
| | | | | |
| | | | | |
| | | | | |

| Area/subjective data | Objective data |
|---|---|
| **Head and Neck** | **Scalp:**<br>• Cleanliness: ______<br>• Abrasions/wound: ______<br>______<br>**Hairs:**<br>• Color: ______<br>• Texture (fine/coarse/brittle/dull): ______<br>• Distribution (hair loss): ______<br>• Dandruff: ______<br>• Pediculi or any other infection: ______<br>**Face (pale, puffiness, expressions, enlargement of parotid glands):** ______<br>______<br>**Neck:**<br>• Lump or mass: ______<br>• Lymphadenopathy: ______<br>• Range of motion (flexion, extension, rotation):<br>______<br>______<br>• Jugular venous pulses: ______<br>**Thyroid gland (landmarks, lump):**<br>______<br>______ |

*Contd...*

| Area/subjective data | Objective data |
|---|---|
| Eyes | **Eyelids:**<br>• Position (ptosis/lid retraction): ____________<br>**Lid margin:**<br>• Edema: ____________<br>• Erythema: ____________<br>• Lesions: ____________<br>**Sclera:**<br>____________<br>____________<br>**Conjunctiva:**<br>____________<br>____________<br>**Pupils:**<br>• Color: ____________<br>• Pupillary response: ____________<br>____________<br>____________<br>**Extraocular movements:**<br>____________<br>____________<br>Use of spectacles/contact lens: ____________<br>____________<br>Visual acuity: ____________<br>____________ |

*Contd...*

| Area/subjective data | Objective data |
|---|---|
| **Ears** | **Use of hearing aids:** ______<br><br>**Auricle (deformity, lesion, discharge, size, symmetry, angle of attachment to head):** ______<br>______<br>______<br>______<br><br>**Mastoid area (tenderness):** ______<br>______<br><br>**External auditory canal (discharge/cerumen/fluid/blood, nodule):** ______<br>______<br><br>**Tympanic membrane (color):** ______<br><br>**Hearing acuity:** ______<br><br>• Whisper test: ______<br><br>• Weber test: ______<br><br>• Rinne test: ______ |

*Contd...*

| Area/subjective data | Objective data |
|---|---|
| **Nose and Sinuses** | **External nose:**<br>• Lesions: __________<br>• Asymmetry: __________<br>• Inflammation: __________<br>**Internal structures of nose:**<br>• Nasal mucosa (color/swelling/exudates/bleeding/polyps):<br>__________<br>__________<br>__________<br>__________<br>Nasal septum (central/deviated): __________<br>**Sinuses:**<br>• Frontal sinuses: __________<br>• Maxillary sinuses: __________ |
| **Mouth and Pharynx** | Lips (symmetry, color, dry/moist):<br>__________<br>Buccal mucosa (color/consistency/lesion/mass):<br>__________<br>Gums (color/lesions/swelling/bleeding/discharge):<br>__________<br>Odor from the mouth: __________<br>Teeth (total number of teeth, color, tooth decay):<br>__________<br>Tongue (symmetry/color/texture/moisture): __________<br>Hard and soft palate (color/lesion):<br>__________<br>Uvula (position/color):<br>__________<br>Tonsils (color/size/exudate):<br>__________<br>Pharynx (color/lesion/exudate):<br>__________ |

*Contd...*

| Area/subjective data | Objective data |
|---|---|
| **Thorax/Lungs** | **Is client on: Room air/oxygen/ventilator**<br>If on oxygen support:<br>• Flow rate: ______<br>• Mode: ______<br>Endotracheal tube: Present/absent: ______<br>**Thorax:**<br>• Shape and symmetry: ______<br>• Position of sternum: ______<br>• Use of accessory muscles: ______<br>• Intercostal space (retraction/bulging): ______<br>• Respiratory rate: ______ Rhythm: ______<br>**Dyspnea (shortness of breath):**<br>• On rest: ______<br>• On exertion: ______<br>• Orthopnea: ______<br>• With expiratory/inspiratory wheezing: ______<br>**Cough:**<br>• Character (dry/hacking/brassy/wheezing): ______<br>• Time (morning/night): ______<br>**Sputum:**<br>• Color (colorless/yellowish/rust color/bright red/black):<br>______<br>• Odor: ______<br>**Chest pain:**<br>• Location (left/right side): ______<br>• Sharp/stabbing/intermittent/dull/aching/persistent: ______<br>• Duration: ______<br>**Wheezing:**<br>• Heard with/without stethoscope: ______<br>Hemoptysis: ______<br>Abnormal breath sounds (crackles/wheezing): ______<br>**Trachea (position, mass):**<br>______<br>______<br>______ |

*Contd...*

| Area/subjective data | Objective data |
|---|---|
| **Heart** | Chest pain: ____________<br>____________<br>• Referred pain (radiates to neck/arm/jaw/shoulders/hands/back/abdomen): ____________<br>____________<br>Palpitations: ____________<br>Heart sounds: ____________<br>Murmurs: ____________ |
| **Breast and Axilla** | **Breast:**<br>• Size and symmetry: ____________<br>• Color: ____________<br>• Venous pattern: ____________<br>• Thickening/edema: ____________<br>• Ulceration/rashes: ____________<br>• Scar: ____________<br>**Areola:**<br>• Color: ____________<br>• Lesion: ____________<br>**Nipple:**<br>• Discharge: ____________<br>• Retraction: ____________<br>• Lesion: ____________<br>**Axilla:**<br>• Tenderness: ____________<br>• Axillary lymph nodes: ____________ |

*Contd...*

| Area/subjective data | Objective data |
|---|---|
| **Abdomen** | Abdominal girth: ______<br>Scars/lesions/rashes: ______<br>Symmetry: ______<br>Abdominal contour: ______<br>Vomiting: ______<br>______<br>______<br>**Changes in bowel habits and stool characteristics:** ______<br>• Diarrhea: ______<br>• Constipation: ______<br>**Bowel sounds (normal/hypoactive/hyperactive/absent):** ______<br>______<br>**Tympany or dullness (during percussion):** ______<br>______<br>______<br>Ascites: ______<br>**Tenderness or swelling:**<br>• All quadrants: ______<br>• Liver: ______<br>• Spleen: ______<br>• Appendix: ______<br>• Kidney: ______<br>• Urinary bladder: ______ |

*Contd...*

| Area/subjective data | Objective data |
|---|---|
| **Genitalia** | Urinary catheter: Present/absent: ________<br>Urination (frequency, amount, color): ________<br>Urinary pattern (urgency, retention): ________<br>Burning micturition: ________<br>Hematuria: ________<br>**Male genitalia:**<br>• Penis: ________<br>• Scrotum: ________<br>• Inguinal area: ________<br>**Female genitalia:**<br>• Mons pubis: ________<br>• Labia majora: ________<br>• Urethra: ________<br>• Vagina: ________<br>• Cervix: ________ |
| **Anus and Rectum** | **Anus:**<br>• Anal opening area (redness, rashes, lump, ulcer, lesion, fissure, hemorrhoids): ________<br>________<br>Rectum (tenderness, smoothness, nodules): ________<br>________ |

*Contd...*

| Area/subjective data | Objective data |
|---|---|
| **Extremities** | Immobility: ____________<br>Coordination: ____________<br>Symmetry: ____________<br>Capillary refill time: ____________<br>Nails (cleanliness, color, clubbing, cyanosis): ____________<br>____________<br>____________<br>Edema: ____________<br>**Range of motion:**<br>• **Shoulder and arm:**<br>Flexion and hyperextension: ____________<br>Adduction and abduction: ____________<br>External and internal rotation: ____________<br>• **Elbows:**<br>Flexion and extension: ____________<br>Supination and pronation: ____________<br>External and internal rotation: ____________<br>• **Wrist:**<br>Flexion and extension: ____________<br>• **Hands and fingers:**<br>Abduction and adduction: ____________<br>Flexion and hyperextension: ____________<br>• **Hips:**<br>Abduction and adduction: ____________<br>Flexion and hyperextension: ____________<br>• **Knees:**<br>Flexion and hyperextension: ____________<br>• **Ankles and feet:**<br>Dorsiflexion and plantar flexion: ____________<br>Eversion and inversion: ____________<br>Abduction and adduction: ____________<br>Varicose veins: ____________ |

*Contd...*

| Area/subjective data | Objective data |
|---|---|
| **Skin** | **Color changes:**<br>• Pallor: ______<br>• Jaundice: ______<br>• Cyanosis: ______<br>Temperature (warm/normal/cold and clammy): ______<br>______<br>Skin texture (rough/smooth): ______<br>Skin turgor: ______<br>Skin integrity (intact/bedsores): ______<br>______<br>Edema: ______<br>Rash (location, itching): ______<br>Lesions (macule/papule/vesicle/nodule/pustule/scar): ______<br>______ |

## LABORATORY INVESTIGATIONS

| Date | Investigations | Patient's Value | Normal Value | Remarks |
|---|---|---|---|---|
| | | | | |

**Radiological investigations:**

Date:________________

Findings: ________________________________________

## MEDICATION

| Trade Name | Pharmaceutical Name | Dose | Route | Frequency | Action |
|---|---|---|---|---|---|
| | | | | | |

## INTAKE AND OUTPUT CHART

Date:___________/___________/___________

| Time | Intake (in mL) | | | | Total | Time | Output (in mL) | | | | | Total |
|---|---|---|---|---|---|---|---|---|---|---|---|---|
| | Oral | IV | NG | Blood | | | Urine | Stool | NG aspiration | Vomiting | Drainage | |
| | | | | | | | | | | | | |
| | | | | | | | | | | | | |
| | | | | | | | | | | | | |
| | | | | | | | | | | | | |
| | | | | | | | | | | | | |
| | | | | | | | | | | | | |
| | | | | | | | | | | | | |
| | | | | | | | | | | | | |
| | | | | | | | | | | | | |
| | | | | | | | | | | | | |
| | | | | | | | | | | | | |
| | | | | | | | | | | | | |
| | | | | | | | | | | | | |
| | | | | | | | | | | | | |
| | | | | | | | | | | | | |
| | | | | | | | | | | | | |
| | | | | | | | | | | | | |
| | | | | | | | | | | | | |
| | | | | | | | | | | | | |
| | | | | | | | | | | | | |
| | | | | | | | | | | | | |
| | | | | | | | | | | | | |
| | | | | | | | | | | | | |
| | | | | | | | | | | | | |
| Total intake (in mL) | | | | | | Total output (in mL) | | | | | | |

Balance: +/– ___________________________

## NURSING MANAGEMENT

**Identified nursing needs and problems of patient:**

**Nursing diagnosis:**

**Short-term goals:**

**Long-term goals:**

## NURSING CARE PLAN

| Assessment (subjective and objective) | Nursing diagnosis | Goal | Planning | Implementation | Rationale | Evaluation |
|---|---|---|---|---|---|---|
| | | | | | | |

| Assessment (subjective and objective) | Nursing diagnosis | Goal | Planning | Implementation | Rationale | Evaluation |
|---|---|---|---|---|---|---|
| | | | | | | |

| Assessment (subjective and objective) | Nursing diagnosis | Goal | Planning | Implementation | Rationale | Evaluation |
| --- | --- | --- | --- | --- | --- | --- |
| | | | | | | |

| Assessment (subjective and objective) | Nursing diagnosis | Goal | Planning | Implementation | Rationale | Evaluation |
|---|---|---|---|---|---|---|
| | | | | | | |

| Assessment (subjective and objective) | Nursing diagnosis | Goal | Planning | Implementation | Rationale | Evaluation |
|---|---|---|---|---|---|---|
| | | | | | | |

| Assessment (subjective and objective) | Nursing diagnosis | Goal | Planning | Implementation | Rationale | Evaluation |
|---|---|---|---|---|---|---|
| | | | | | | |

## HEALTH EDUCATION

1. **Disease Condition**

2. **Personal Hygiene**

3. **Diet**

4. **Lifestyle Modification**

5. **Medication**

6. **Follow-up Care**

## EVALUATION CRITERIA FOR NURSING CARE PLAN

Name of the Student: ____________________

Diagnosis of Patient: ____________________

Ward/Unit: ____________________ Date of Submission: ____________________

| Sl. No. | Evaluation Criteria | Marks Obtained | Maximum Marks |
|---|---|---|---|
| 1 | Utilized therapeutic communication skills while interacting with patient and his/her family members | | 2 |
| 2 | Patient history | | 5 |
| 3 | Subjective and objective assessment | | 5 |
| 4 | Prioritized nursing diagnosis | | 2 |
| 5 | Goals | | 2 |
| 6 | Planning | | 2 |
| 7 | Implementation with rationale | | 2 |
| 8 | Evaluation | | 2 |
| 9 | Health education | | 2 |
| 10 | Timely submission | | 1 |
| **Total marks** | | | **25** |

**Remarks:** ____________________

____________________

____________________

**Signature of the Student**

**Signature of the Clinical Supervisor**

**Date:** ____________________

**Date:** ____________________

# NURSING CARE PLAN–4

Date of collection of health history: _________ / _________ / _________

## I. BIOGRAPHICAL DATA OF THE PATIENT

Name of the patient: ______________________________

Fathers/Husband's name: ______________________________

Age: ____________________ Gender: Male/Female ____________________

Hospital: ______________________________

C.R./IP No.: ______________ Ward: ______________ Bed No.: ______________

Educational status: ____________________ Occupation: ____________________

Religion: ____________________ Marital status: ____________________

Address: ______________________________

______________________________

Date of admission: ______________________________

Treatment under Dr.: ______________________________

Diagnosis: ______________________________

Surgery performed, if any: ______________________________

Date of surgery performed: ______________________________

## II. CHIEF COMPLAINTS

At the time of admission: ______________________________

At present:

## III. HISTORY OF PRESENT ILLNESS

(Includes details about chief complaints: Character, onset-sudden/gradual, location, duration, severity, pattern, aggravating factors, relieving factors, associated manifestations)

## IV. PAST HEALTH HISTORY

(a) Childhood illness: ______________________________

______________________________

(b) Adult illnesses: ______________________________

______________________________

(c) Psychiatric illnesses: ______________________________

______________________________

(d) Previous hospitalizations: ______________________________

______________________________

______________________________

(e) Previous surgical or diagnostic procedures: ______________________________

______________________________

(f) Allergies to foods/medications: ______________________________

______________________________

(g) Menstrual history (for female patient):

Last menstrual period (LMP) ______________ Menopausal: Yes/No ______________

Age at menarche: ______________ years. Menstruation: Regular/irregular duration: ______________

Does bleeding/spotting occur between periods: Yes/No ______________

Is pain associated with periods: ______________

(h) Past obstetrical history:

Have never been pregnant: ______________

Birth control/contraception: ______________

| **Number of pregnancies** | **Year** | **Pregnancy** (normal/miscarriage/abortion) | **Delivery** (normal/assisted/ cesarean section) | **Gender of baby** | **Puerperium** (normal/ complicated) |
|---|---|---|---|---|---|
| | | | | | |
| | | | | | |
| | | | | | |
| | | | | | |
| | | | | | |

## V. FAMILY HISTORY

(a) Family composition:

| Name | Age | Gender | Relationship with patient | Educational status | Occupation | Income | Health status |
|---|---|---|---|---|---|---|---|
| | | | | | | | |

(b) Family tree/genogram:

Key:

Male ○

Female □

Patient →

Deceased ■ ●

(c) History of any recent death in family: Yes/No

Relationship with patient: ________________ Age at death: ________________

Cause of death: ________________________________

(d) History of any chronic illness in family:

(Hypertension, heart disease, diabetes, tuberculosis, asthma, renal disorder, arthritis, cancer, allergies, epilepsy, mental illness, etc.): Yes/No

If yes, give details: ________________________________

________________________________

________________________________

(e) History of any communicable disease in family: ______________________

______________________

______________________

(f) History of any hereditary disease in family: ______________________

______________________

______________________

## VI. LIFESTYLE

(a) Diet: Vegetarian/eggetarian/nonvegetarian/special diet: ______________________

______________________

(b) Bowel and bladder habit: ______________________

______________________

(c) Use of any addictive or illicit substance/drug (heroine/cocaine/alcohol/tobacco): Yes/No

______________________

______________________

______________________

______________________

(d) Sleeping pattern: ______________________

______________________

(e) Exercise: ______________________

______________________

(f) Recreation: ______________________

______________________

(g) Religious belief: ______________________

______________________

## VII. ENVIRONMENTAL HISTORY

(a) Physical-type of housing: ______________________________

______________________________

(b) Environmental hygiene: ______________________________

______________________________

(c) Source of drinking water: ______________________________

______________________________

(d) Presence of flies/mosquitoes/rodents: ______________________________

______________________________

(e) Disposal of excreta: ______________________________

______________________________

(f) Environmental pollution: ______________________________

______________________________

(g) Exposure to hazardous waste: ______________________________

______________________________

# GENERAL PHYSICAL EXAMINATION

## I. GENERAL APPEARANCE

Level of consciousness (conscious/semiconscious/unconscious/coma): ____________________

Orientation (time, place and person): ____________________

____________________

____________________

Activity (active/dull): ____________________

Body built (average/thin/obese): ____________________

Look (anxious/depressed): ____________________

Posture (Body curves: Lordosis/kyphosis/scoliosis): ____________________

## II. ANTHROPOMETRIC MEASUREMENT

Height: ____________ Weight: ____________ BMI: ____________

[Body mass index; BMI = Weight (in kilograms)/Height$^2$ (in meters)]

## III. VITAL SIGNS

| Date/vitals | Temperature (in C°/F°) | Pulse (beats/min) | Respiration (breaths/min) | Blood pressure (in mm Hg) |
|---|---|---|---|---|
| | | | | |
| | | | | |
| | | | | |
| | | | | |
| | | | | |
| | | | | |
| | | | | |

| Area/subjective data | Objective data |
|---|---|
| **Head and Neck** | **Scalp:**<br>• Cleanliness: ____________<br>• Abrasions/wound: ____________<br>____________<br>**Hairs:**<br>• Color: ____________<br>• Texture (fine/coarse/brittle/dull): ____________<br>• Distribution (hair loss): ____________<br>• Dandruff: ____________<br>• Pediculi or any other infection: ____________<br>**Face (pale, puffiness, expressions, enlargement of parotid glands):** ____________<br>____________<br>**Neck:**<br>• Lump or mass: ____________<br>• Lymphadenopathy: ____________<br>• Range of motion (flexion, extension, rotation):<br>____________<br>____________<br>• Jugular venous pulses: ____________<br>**Thyroid gland (landmarks, lump):**<br>____________<br>____________ |

*Contd...*

| Area/subjective data | Objective data |
|---|---|
| Eyes | **Eyelids:**<br>• Position (ptosis/lid retraction): ____________<br>**Lid margin:**<br>• Edema: ____________<br>• Erythema: ____________<br>• Lesions: ____________<br>**Sclera:**<br>____________<br>____________<br>**Conjunctiva:**<br>____________<br>____________<br>**Pupils:**<br>• Color: ____________<br>• Pupillary response: ____________<br>____________<br>____________<br>**Extraocular movements:**<br>____________<br>____________<br>Use of spectacles/contact lens: ____________<br>____________<br>Visual acuity: ____________<br>____________ |

*Contd...*

| Area/subjective data | Objective data |
|---|---|
| **Ears** | **Use of hearing aids:** ____________<br><br>**Auricle (deformity, lesion, discharge, size, symmetry, angle of attachment to head):** ____________<br>____________<br>____________<br>____________<br><br>**Mastoid area (tenderness):** ____________<br>____________<br><br>**External auditory canal (discharge/cerumen/fluid/blood, nodule):** ____________<br>____________<br><br>**Tympanic membrane (color):** ____________<br><br>**Hearing acuity:** ____________<br><br>• Whisper test: ____________<br><br>• Weber test: ____________<br><br>• Rinne test: ____________ |

*Contd...*

| Area/subjective data | Objective data |
|---|---|
| **Nose and Sinuses** | **External nose:**<br>• Lesions: ________<br>• Asymmetry: ________<br>• Inflammation: ________<br>**Internal structures of nose:**<br>• Nasal mucosa (color/swelling/exudates/bleeding/polyps):<br>________<br>________<br>________<br>________<br>Nasal septum (central/deviated): ________<br>**Sinuses:**<br>• Frontal sinuses: ________<br>• Maxillary sinuses: ________ |
| **Mouth and Pharynx** | Lips (symmetry, color, dry/moist):<br>________<br>Buccal mucosa (color/consistency/lesion/mass):<br>________<br>Gums (color/lesions/swelling/bleeding/discharge):<br>________<br>Odor from the mouth: ________<br>Teeth (total number of teeth, color, tooth decay):<br>________<br>Tongue (symmetry/color/texture/moisture): ________<br>Hard and soft palate (color/lesion):<br>________<br>Uvula (position/color):<br>________<br>Tonsils (color/size/exudate):<br>________<br>Pharynx (color/lesion/exudate):<br>________ |

*Contd...*

| Area/subjective data | Objective data |
|---|---|
| **Thorax/Lungs** | **Is client on: Room air/oxygen/ventilator**<br>If on oxygen support:<br>• Flow rate: ______<br>• Mode: ______<br>Endotracheal tube: Present/absent: ______<br>**Thorax:**<br>• Shape and symmetry: ______<br>• Position of sternum: ______<br>• Use of accessory muscles: ______<br>• Intercostal space (retraction/bulging): ______<br>• Respiratory rate: ______ Rhythm: ______<br>**Dyspnea (shortness of breath):**<br>• On rest: ______<br>• On exertion: ______<br>• Orthopnea: ______<br>• With expiratory/inspiratory wheezing: ______<br>**Cough:**<br>• Character (dry/hacking/brassy/wheezing): ______<br>• Time (morning/night): ______<br>**Sputum:**<br>• Color (colorless/yellowish/rust color/bright red/black):<br>______<br>• Odor: ______<br>**Chest pain:**<br>• Location (left/right side): ______<br>• Sharp/stabbing/intermittent/dull/aching/persistent: ______<br>• Duration: ______<br>**Wheezing:**<br>• Heard with/without stethoscope: ______<br>Hemoptysis: ______<br>Abnormal breath sounds (crackles/wheezing): ______<br>**Trachea (position, mass):**<br>______<br>______<br>______ |

*Contd...*

| Area/subjective data | Objective data |
|---|---|
| **Heart** | Chest pain: ____________________<br>____________________<br>• Referred pain (radiates to neck/arm/jaw/shoulders/hands/back/abdomen): ____________<br>____________________<br>Palpitations: ____________________<br>Heart sounds: ____________________<br>Murmurs: ____________________ |
| **Breast and Axilla** | **Breast:**<br>• Size and symmetry: ____________________<br>• Color: ____________________<br>• Venous pattern: ____________________<br>• Thickening/edema: ____________________<br>• Ulceration/rashes: ____________________<br>• Scar: ____________________<br>**Areola:**<br>• Color: ____________________<br>• Lesion: ____________________<br>**Nipple:**<br>• Discharge: ____________________<br>• Retraction: ____________________<br>• Lesion: ____________________<br>**Axilla:**<br>• Tenderness: ____________________<br>• Axillary lymph nodes: ____________________ |

*Contd...*

| Area/subjective data | Objective data |
|---|---|
| **Abdomen** | Abdominal girth: ______<br>Scars/lesions/rashes: ______<br>Symmetry: ______<br>Abdominal contour: ______<br>Vomiting: ______<br>______<br>______<br>**Changes in bowel habits and stool characteristics:** ______<br>• Diarrhea: ______<br>• Constipation: ______<br>**Bowel sounds (normal/hypoactive/hyperactive/absent):** ______<br>______<br>**Tympany or dullness (during percussion):** ______<br>______<br>______<br>Ascites: ______<br>**Tenderness or swelling:**<br>• All quadrants: ______<br>• Liver: ______<br>• Spleen: ______<br>• Appendix: ______<br>• Kidney: ______<br>• Urinary bladder: ______ |

*Contd...*

| Area/subjective data | Objective data |
|---|---|
| **Genitalia** | Urinary catheter: Present/absent: ________<br>Urination (frequency, amount, color): ________<br>Urinary pattern (urgency, retention): ________<br>Burning micturition: ________<br>Hematuria: ________<br>**Male genitalia:**<br>• Penis: ________<br>• Scrotum: ________<br>• Inguinal area: ________<br>**Female genitalia:**<br>• Mons pubis: ________<br>• Labia majora: ________<br>• Urethra: ________<br>• Vagina: ________<br>• Cervix: ________ |
| **Anus and Rectum** | **Anus:**<br>• Anal opening area (redness, rashes, lump, ulcer, lesion, fissure, hemorrhoids): ________<br>________<br>Rectum (tenderness, smoothness, nodules): ________<br>________ |

*Contd...*

| Area/subjective data | Objective data |
|---|---|
| **Extremities** | Immobility: ______<br>Coordination: ______<br>Symmetry: ______<br>Capillary refill time: ______<br>Nails (cleanliness, color, clubbing, cyanosis): ______<br>______<br>______<br>Edema: ______<br>**Range of motion:**<br>• **Shoulder and arm:**<br>Flexion and hyperextension: ______<br>Adduction and abduction: ______<br>External and internal rotation: ______<br>• **Elbows:**<br>Flexion and extension: ______<br>Supination and pronation: ______<br>External and internal rotation: ______<br>• **Wrist:**<br>Flexion and extension: ______<br>• **Hands and fingers:**<br>Abduction and adduction: ______<br>Flexion and hyperextension: ______<br>• **Hips:**<br>Abduction and adduction: ______<br>Flexion and hyperextension: ______<br>• **Knees:**<br>Flexion and hyperextension: ______<br>• **Ankles and feet:**<br>Dorsiflexion and plantar flexion: ______<br>Eversion and inversion: ______<br>Abduction and adduction: ______<br>Varicose veins: ______ |

*Contd...*

| Area/subjective data | Objective data |
|---|---|
| **Skin** | **Color changes:**<br>• Pallor: ________<br>• Jaundice: ________<br>• Cyanosis: ________<br>Temperature (warm/normal/cold and clammy): ________<br>________<br>Skin texture (rough/smooth): ________<br>Skin turgor: ________<br>Skin integrity (intact/bedsores): ________<br>________<br>Edema: ________<br>Rash (location, itching): ________<br>Lesions (macule/papule/vesicle/nodule/pustule/scar): ________<br>________ |

## LABORATORY INVESTIGATIONS

| Date | Investigations | Patient's Value | Normal Value | Remarks |
|---|---|---|---|---|
| | | | | |

**Radiological investigations:**

Date:________________

Findings: ________________________________________________

## MEDICATION

| Trade Name | Pharmaceutical Name | Dose | Route | Frequency | Action |
|---|---|---|---|---|---|
| | | | | | |

## INTAKE AND OUTPUT CHART

Date:__________/__________/__________

| Time | Intake (in mL) | | | | Total | Time | Output (in mL) | | | | | Total |
|---|---|---|---|---|---|---|---|---|---|---|---|---|
| | Oral | IV | NG | Blood | | | Urine | Stool | NG aspiration | Vomiting | Drainage | |
| | | | | | | | | | | | | |
| | | | | | | | | | | | | |
| | | | | | | | | | | | | |
| | | | | | | | | | | | | |
| | | | | | | | | | | | | |
| | | | | | | | | | | | | |
| | | | | | | | | | | | | |
| | | | | | | | | | | | | |
| | | | | | | | | | | | | |
| | | | | | | | | | | | | |
| | | | | | | | | | | | | |
| | | | | | | | | | | | | |
| | | | | | | | | | | | | |
| | | | | | | | | | | | | |
| | | | | | | | | | | | | |
| | | | | | | | | | | | | |
| | | | | | | | | | | | | |
| | | | | | | | | | | | | |
| | | | | | | | | | | | | |
| | | | | | | | | | | | | |
| | | | | | | | | | | | | |
| | | | | | | | | | | | | |
| | | | | | | | | | | | | |
| | | | | | | | | | | | | |
| Total intake (in mL) | | | | | | Total output (in mL) | | | | | | |

Balance: +/– ____________________

## NURSING MANAGEMENT

**Identified nursing needs and problems of patient:**

**Nursing diagnosis:**

**Short-term goals:**

**Long-term goals:**

## NURSING CARE PLAN

| Assessment (subjective and objective) | Nursing diagnosis | Goal | Planning | Implementation | Rationale | Evaluation |
|---|---|---|---|---|---|---|
| | | | | | | |

| Assessment (subjective and objective) | Nursing diagnosis | Goal | Planning | Implementation | Rationale | Evaluation |
|---|---|---|---|---|---|---|
| | | | | | | |

| Assessment (subjective and objective) | Nursing diagnosis | Goal | Planning | Implementation | Rationale | Evaluation |
|---|---|---|---|---|---|---|
| | | | | | | |

| Assessment (subjective and objective) | Nursing diagnosis | Goal | Planning | Implementation | Rationale | Evaluation |
| --- | --- | --- | --- | --- | --- | --- |
| | | | | | | |

| Assessment (subjective and objective) | Nursing diagnosis | Goal | Planning | Implementation | Rationale | Evaluation |
|---|---|---|---|---|---|---|
| | | | | | | |

| Assessment (subjective and objective) | Nursing diagnosis | Goal | Planning | Implementation | Rationale | Evaluation |
|---|---|---|---|---|---|---|
| | | | | | | |

## HEALTH EDUCATION

1. **Disease Condition**

2. **Personal Hygiene**

3. **Diet**

4. **Lifestyle Modification**

5. **Medication**

6. **Follow-up Care**